Bountiful Bariatric Recipes

A Complete Cookbook of Stage 4 Dish Ideas!

BY: Allie Allen

COOK & ENJOY

Copyright 2020 Allie Allen

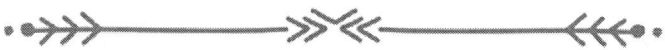

Copyright Notes

This book is written as an informational tool. While the author has taken every precaution to ensure the accuracy of the information provided therein, the reader is warned that they assume all risk when following the content. The author will not be held responsible for any damages that may occur as a result of the readers' actions.

The author does not give permission to reproduce this book in any form, including but not limited to: print, social media posts, electronic copies or photocopies, unless permission is expressly given in writing.

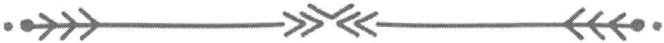

Table of Contents

Introduction 6

Bariatric Breakfast Recipes 8

   1 – Breakfast Fritters 9

   2 – Baked Ham & Egg Cups 11

   3 – Lime & Avocado Omelet 13

   4 – Crustless Spinach & Turkey Quiche 15

   5 – Apricot Oatmeal 18

Bariatric Recipes for Lunch, Dinner, Side Dishes and Appetizers 20

   6 – Indian Veggie Skillet 21

   7 – Chicken Soup 23

   8 – Curried Potatoes 25

   9 – Beef Avocado Stir Fry 27

   10 – Avocado Chickpea Salad 29

   11 – Chicken Cacciatore 31

   12 – Chicken Tortilla Soup 33

   13 – Turkey Chili 35

14 – Sausage & Summer Beans 37

15 – Rosemary Lemon Chicken 39

16 – Couscous & Veggies 41

17 – Squash Soup 43

18 – Turkey Cabbage Rolls 45

19 – Tofu Salad 48

20 – Apple & Pork Stew 50

21 – Stuffed Apple Pork Chops 53

22 – Chicken Salad with Pecans & Apples 55

23 – Cauliflower Bake 57

24 – Steak Fajitas 59

25 – Chicken Lentil Soup 62

26 – Flounder & Roasted Vegetables 64

27 – French Onion & Leek Soup 66

28 – Turkey Taco Casserole 68

Bariatric Dessert Recipes 70

29 – Butterscotch Dessert Bars 71

30 – Cinnamon Pear 74

4

31 – Berry Cobbler 76

32 – Peanut Butter Bites 78

33 – Skinny Brownies 80

Conclusion 82

About the Author 83

Author's Afterthoughts 85

Introduction

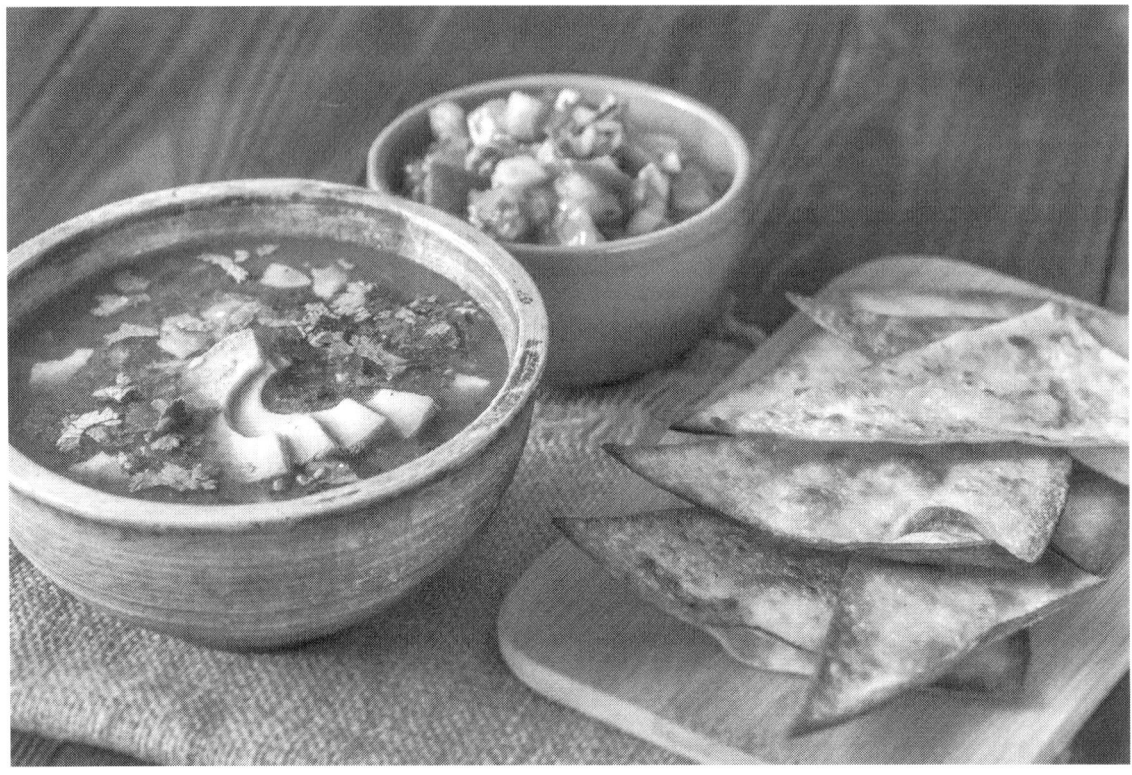

When you get to phase 4 of your bariatric diet, how similar will the foods be to your old diet?

Can you still eat the types of foods you used to eat?

Can you make meals that your family will enjoy, too?

Phase 4 comes after you've been drinking fluids and eating gelatin-type foods for a while. By the time you reach this phase, you'll be tired of smooth foods and liquids and ready to move toward more "normal" food textures.

You'll want to be careful to ensure that your portions contain small bite-sized pieces, but you can also add flavors and textures that your family will enjoy, too.

Don't be afraid to be creative with phase 4, as long as you don't go overboard with spicy foods or large portions. This is the most satisfying and interesting phase of the bariatric diet if you are creative with the dishes you prepare.

Phase 4 also means eating healthy foods, not the same old fast food that added to your weight and unhealthiness in the first place. You will be able to back off on supplements if you get most of your necessary vitamins and minerals through your diet.

Concentrate on including lean proteins, vegetables, fruits, fat-free dairy products, whole grains & a few healthy fats. Turn the page, and let's start cooking phase 4 dishes…

Bariatric Breakfast Recipes

1 – Breakfast Fritters

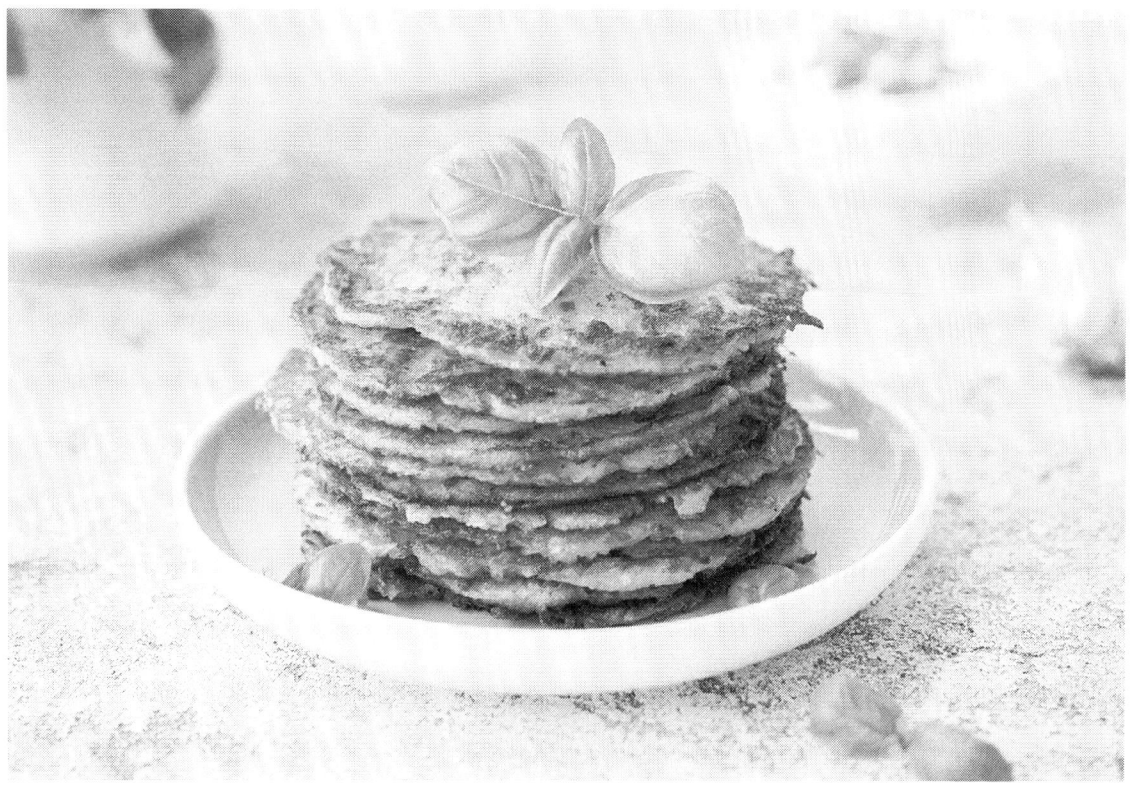

These are not the same as conventional zucchini fritters. They have fewer calories and less fat, but they still can fill you up till lunch time.

Makes 4 Servings

Cooking + Prep Time: 40 minutes

Ingredients:

- 6 eggs, large
- 1/2 cup of quick oats, raw
- 1 grated zucchini, small
- For cooking: oil, olive

Instructions:

Combine eggs, zucchini and oats in mixing bowl. Mix till combined well.

Spray non-stick pan. Ladle batter onto pan like you would with pancakes.

Cook till pancakes (fritters) are done on both sides, watching heat carefully so they are not overcooked. Top with guacamole or hummus. Serve.

2 – Baked Ham & Egg Cups

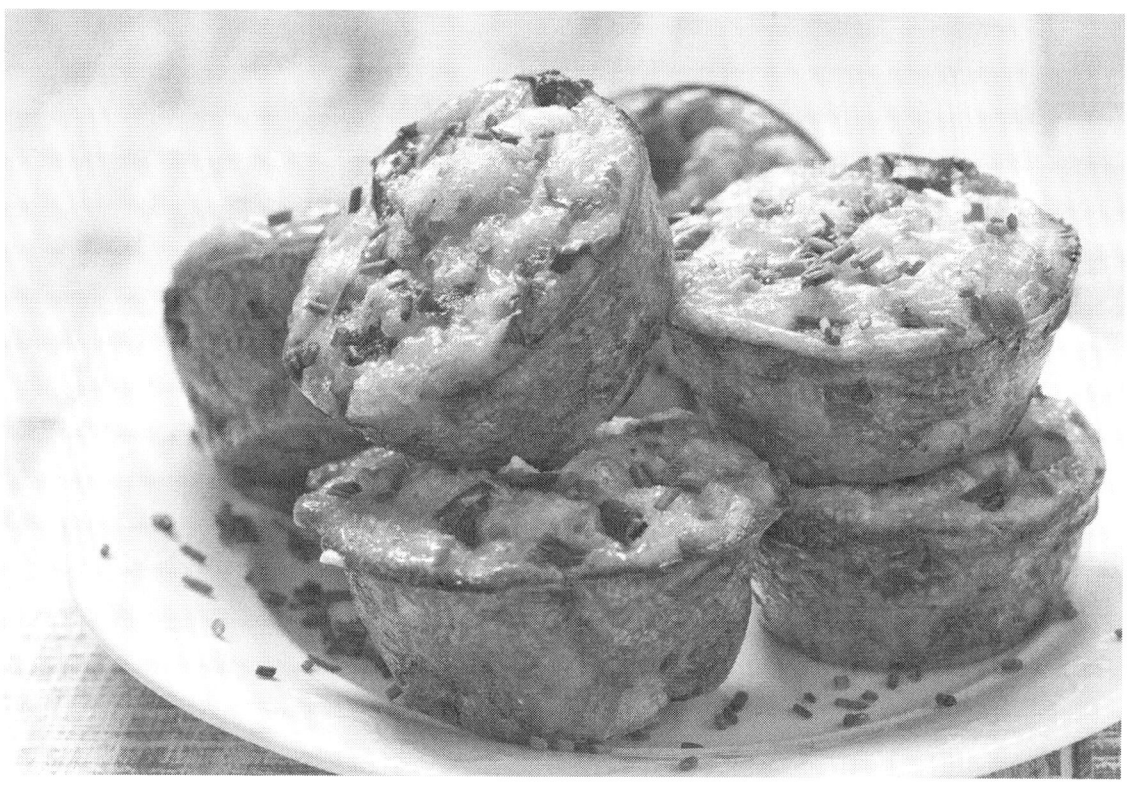

I often prepare eggs in the morning, but some days are more hurried, and we just want to grab something fast. That's where these baked ham & egg cups come in handy since I prepare them ahead of time.

Makes 12 Servings

Cooking + Prep Time: 35 minutes

Ingredients:

- 12 ham slices
- 12 eggs, large
- As desired:
- Salt, kosher
- Pepper, ground
- Paprika, ground

Instructions:

Preheat the oven to 375F.

Line muffin tin cups with ham slices. Crack one egg in each cup. Season as desired. Bake in 375F oven for 20 minutes.

Remove from oven and let them cool for a few minutes. Remove from muffin pans. Serve.

3 – Lime & Avocado Omelet

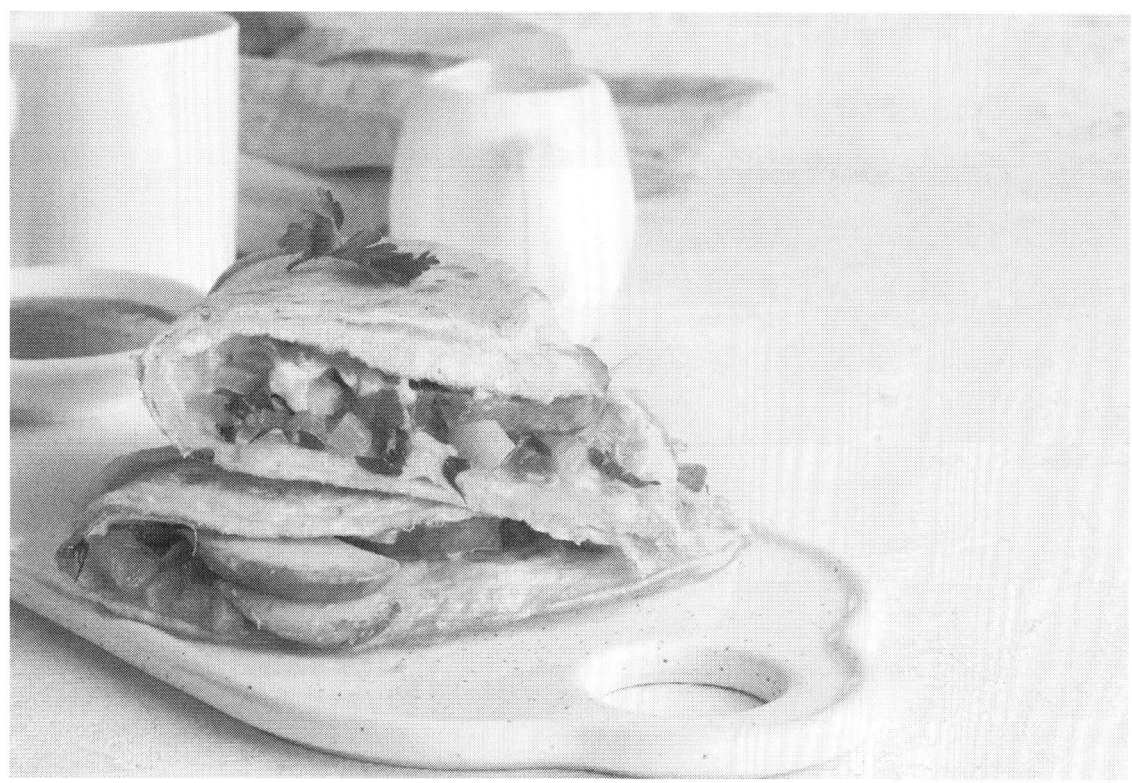

The combinations of these tasty ingredients all together – avocado, eggs, lime, pineapple, bacon, cheese, and more – will have your stomach growling in the morning.

Makes 1-2 Servings

Cooking + Prep Time: 40 minutes

Ingredients:

- 2 or 3 eggs, large
- 1/8 diced medium onion, yellow
- 1-2 chili peppers, mild
- 1/2 tbsp. of ghee or clarified butter
- 1/2 avocado, ripe
- 1/2 lime, fresh juice only
- Salt, kosher, as desired

Instructions:

Melt ghee on med. heat in non-stick, medium or large pan.

Add chilies & diced onions. Season with pinch of kosher salt and sauté till golden.

Whisk eggs in medium bowl. Salt as desired. Add 1/4 of avocado. Smash avocado up like chunky guacamole.

Cut remaining 1/4 avocado in cubes. Place in separate bowl. Squeeze lime juice over it and season as desired.

Add chilies and onions to egg mixture. Combine well.

Melt a bit more ghee in separate pan. Add egg mixture and coat pan evenly.

Cook till it turns light gold in color and base seems solid. Flip and cook the other side.

Slice the omelet on plate. Add cubed avocado over 1/2 of egg. Fold over the other half. Sprinkle with additional fresh lime juice. Serve.

4 – Crustless Spinach & Turkey Quiche

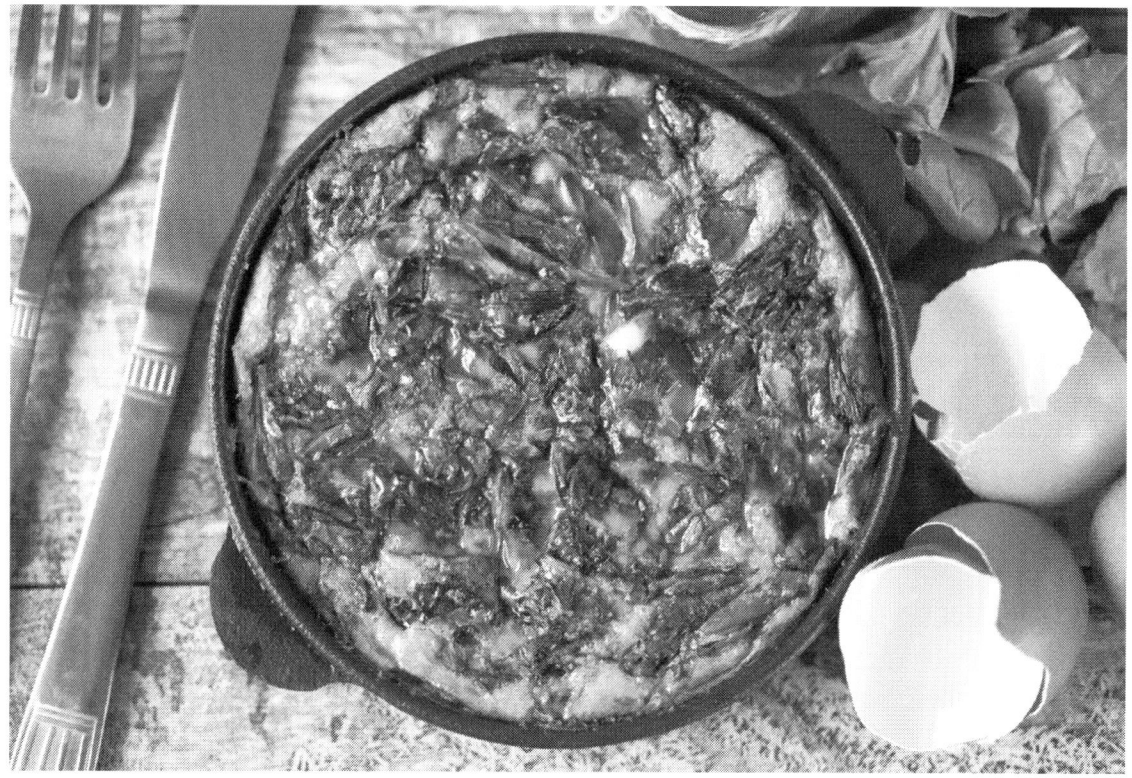

This is a healthier quiche since it omits the crust. I do add a bit of whole wheat flour, which helps to bind its egg mixture together.

Makes 8-12 Servings

Cooking + Prep Time: 55 minutes

Ingredients:

- 3/4 cup of smoked turkey, cubed
- 1/2 cup of onion, chopped
- 1/8 tsp. of pepper, ground
- 3/4 cup of Swiss cheese shreds
- 1 cup leaves of baby spinach, fresh
- 1 cup of cottage cheese, 2%
- 1/2 cup of half 'n half, fat-free
- 1/4 cup of cheddar cheese shreds, reduced-fat
- 2 eggs, large
- 2 egg whites, large
- 1/2 cup of pastry flour, whole wheat
- 1 tsp. of baking powder, pure

Instructions:

Preheat the oven to 350F.

Heat non-stick skillet on med-high. Coat with non-stick spray. Add the turkey, pepper and onions. Sauté for about four minutes, till turkey has browned lightly.

Sprinkle just 1/4 cup of Swiss cheese shreds in 9" pie plate. Top with the turkey mixture.

Combine the remainder of Swiss cheese with spinach and next five ingredients in large mixing bowl. Stir with whisk.

Spoon flour lightly into measuring cup and level using a knife. Combine the flour with baking powder in small bowl and stir with whisk.

Add the flour mixture to the egg mixture and stir till blended well. Pour the mixture over the turkey mixture.

Bake in 350F oven for 45 minutes. When you insert a knife in middle, it should come back clean. Serve.

5 – Apricot Oatmeal

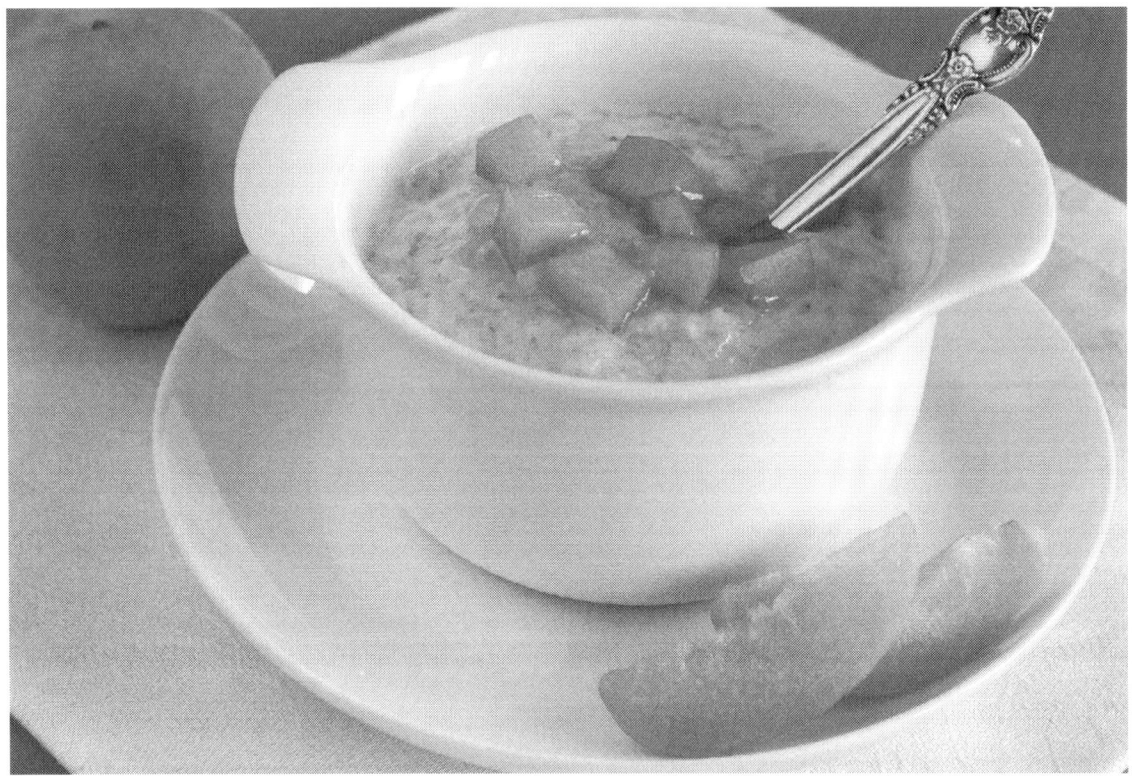

Overnight oats are a simple and tasty way to have your breakfast pretty much ready when you get up. The dry oats and the remaining ingredients are poured into a mug or jar with milk and allowed to set overnight in the fridge.

Makes 1 Serving

Cooking + Prep Time: 45 minutes

Ingredients:

- 1/2 cup of oats, old-fashioned
- 1 tsp. of cinnamon, ground
- 1/4 tsp. of allspice, ground
- 1/4 tsp. of ginger, ground
- 1 tsp. of vanilla extract, pure
- 1/4 cup of dried apricots, chopped
- 1 cup of milk, low fat

Instructions:

Combine the ingredients in covered jar or bowl with a cup of milk the night before.

Place mixture in refrigerator and allow to set overnight.

Serve cold or warm when you get up.

Bariatric Recipes for Lunch, Dinner, Side Dishes and Appetizers

6 – Indian Veggie Skillet

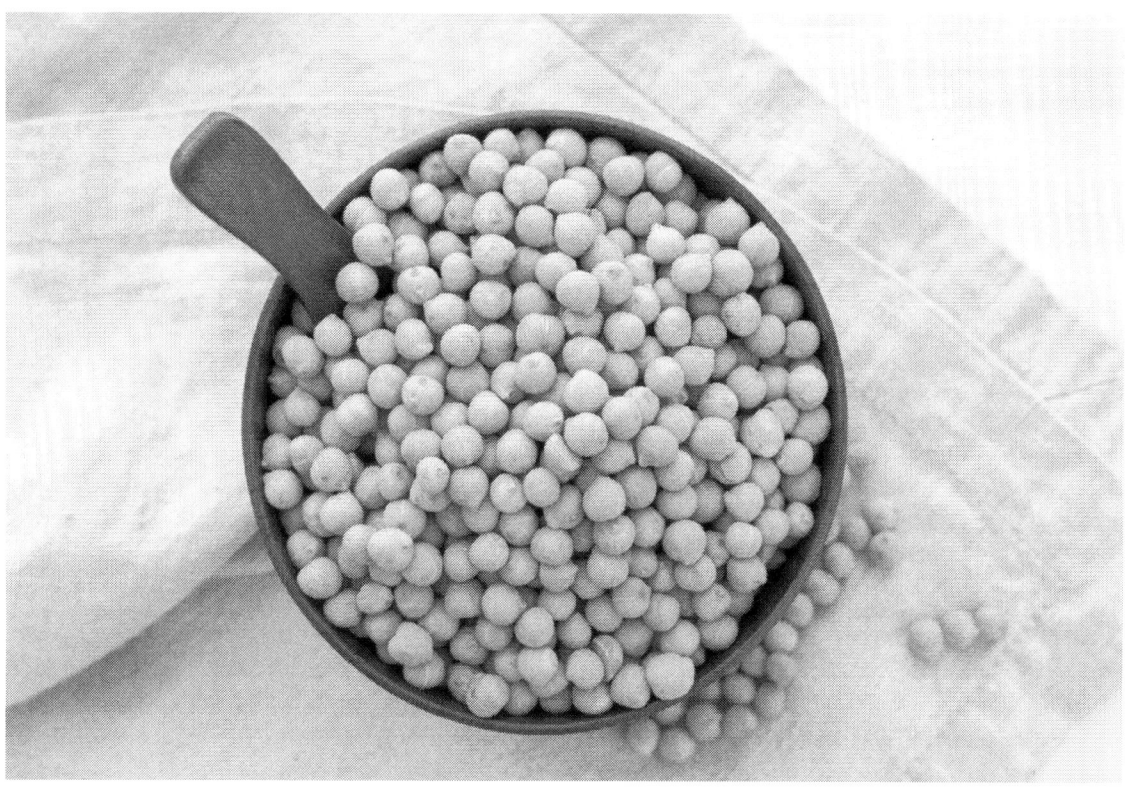

Do you enjoy Indian spices, including ginger or curry? This Indian vegetable recipe is delicious, vegan, gluten-free, and phase 4 post-bariatric surgery suitable.

Makes 4 Servings

Cooking + Prep Time: 1 hour

Ingredients:

- 1 x 14-ounce can of drained, rinsed chickpeas
- 1 & 3/4 cup of water, filtered
- 1 cup of uncooked rice, brown
- 1 cup of mixed vegetables, frozen
- 1/2 tsp. of cumin, ground
- 2 tsp. of oil, olive
- 1 peeled, diced sweet potato, medium
- 1 peeled, diced carrot
- 1 minced garlic clove
- 1/2 diced onion, medium
- Salt, kosher, to taste
- Pepper, ground, to taste

Instructions:

Chop sweet potato, carrot, garlic and onion.

Heat the oil in large-sized skillet on med. heat.

Add cumin and onion. Cook while stirring for a minute.

Add the remainder of ingredients. Bring to boil, then cover. Reduce the heat.

Simmer for 30-35 minutes. Cover pan. Allow to stand for 10-12 minutes and serve hot.

7 – Chicken Soup

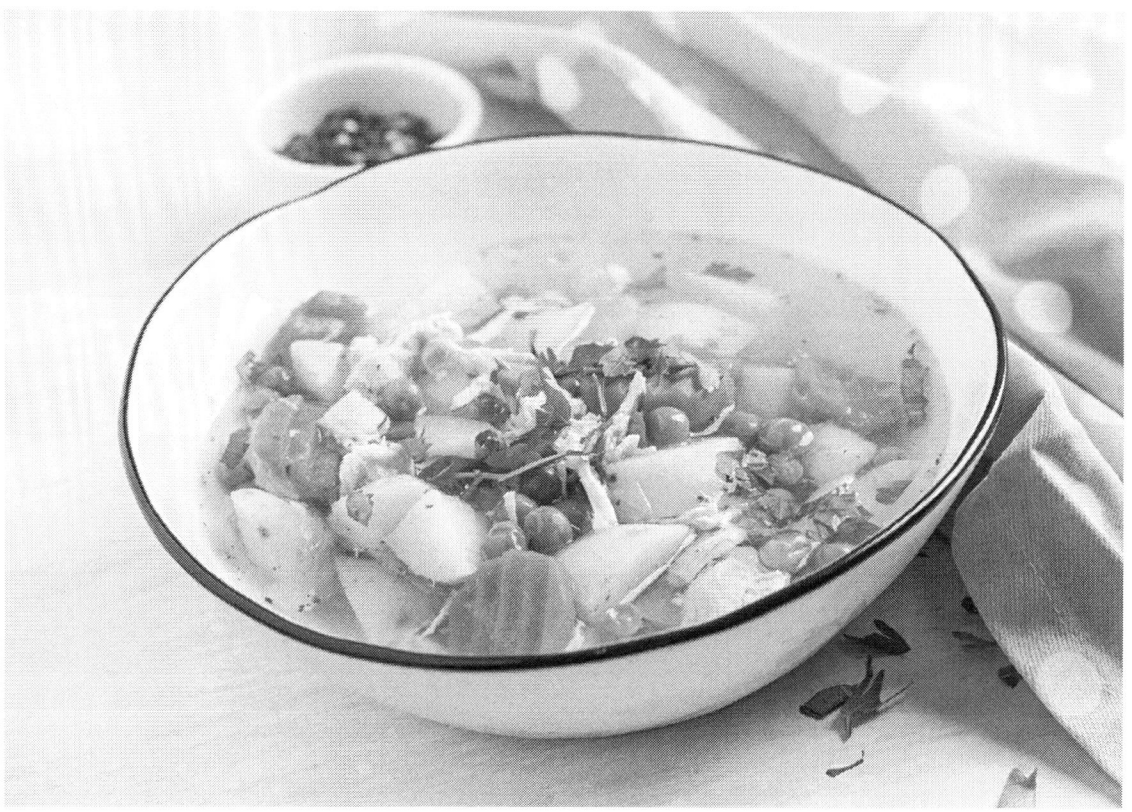

This is one of the first dishes suitable for preparation after bariatric surgery. It's delicious and comforting and has more protein than canned soup. In phase 4, you can include chicken pieces, too, rather than just broth.

Makes 4 Servings

Cooking + Prep Time: 40 minutes

Ingredients:

- 1 tsp. of oil, olive
- 1 & 1/4 pounds of chicken thighs, boneless
- 1 chopped carrot
- 1 chopped celery stalk
- 1/4 cup of onions, chopped
- 3 cups of chicken broth, low sodium
- 1/4 tsp. of rosemary, dried
- 1/4 tsp. of thyme
- Salt, kosher, as desired
- Pepper, ground, as desired

Instructions:

Heat the oil on med. heat in Dutch oven. Add chicken & cook fully through. Remove the chicken and allow to cool. Once you can handle it, cut chicken in small chunks.

Sauté carrot, onions & celery in Dutch oven. Leave the liquid from chicken cooking in the pot, to add to the soup's flavor. Sauté the vegetables for five minutes.

Add rosemary, chicken chunks and broth. Bring to boil. Allow to simmer for 10 to 15 minutes.

Remove pot from heat. Pour soup in blender. Puree till you have the consistency you desire. Serve.

8 – Curried Potatoes

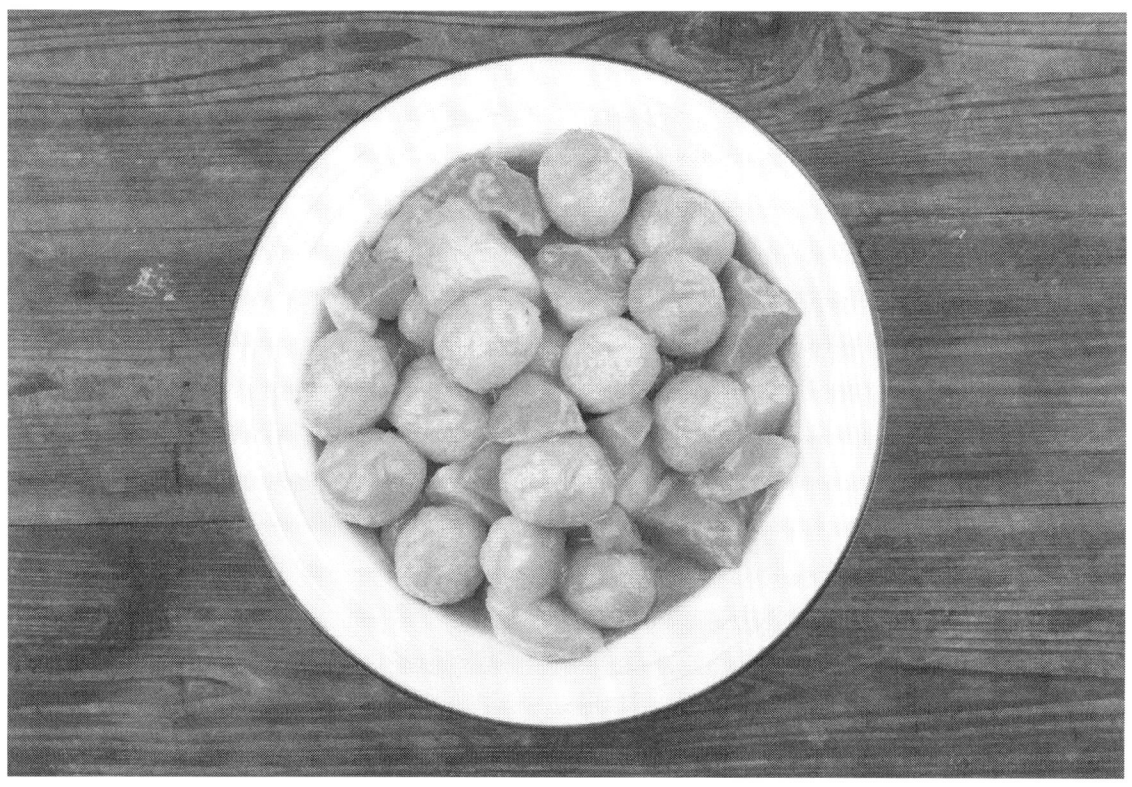

Curry is made from a variety of spices, often including garlic, chili powder, coriander, cumin, and turmeric. You can leave out any spices that may be too strong for your taste.

Makes 4 Servings

Cooking + Prep Time: 50 minutes

Ingredients:

- 1 fresh lemon, juice only
- 1/2 tbsp. of curry powder
- 3/4 cup of chicken broth, low sodium
- 2 x 1" cubed potatoes, medium
- 1 chopped onion, small
- 1/4 cup of oil, olive

Instructions:

Peel, then dice potatoes and onion.

Boil potatoes in pan till soft. Drain water off. Add enough cold water to fully cover potatoes.

Add oil in skillet on med. heat.

Cook onions in oil till they turn yellow.

Drain water from potatoes. Add to skillet.

Add lemon juice, broth and curry powder.

Cook till potatoes absorb broth and serve.

9 – Beef Avocado Stir Fry

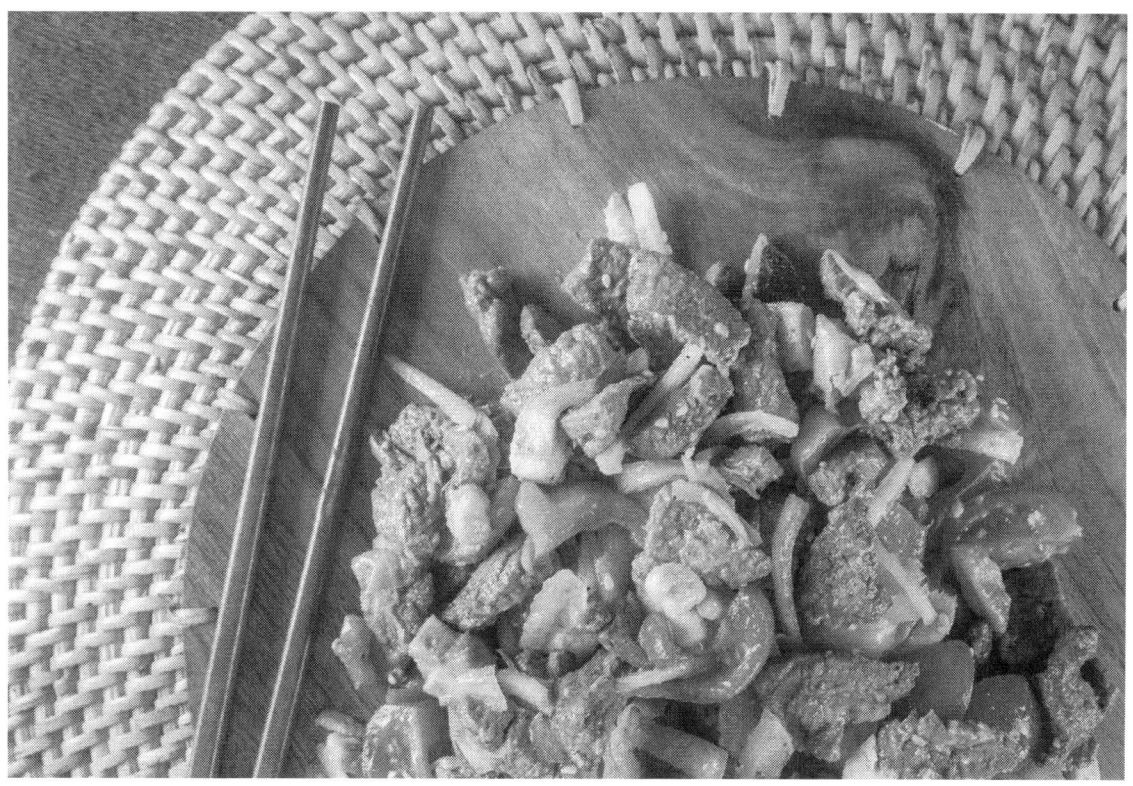

Once the beef is tolerable after bariatric surgery, this recipe may become a favorite. It's simple to make and tastes great reheated, too.

Makes 4 Servings

Cooking + Prep Time: 35 minutes

Ingredients:

- 1 peeled, cubed avocado
- 1 & 1/2 tbsp. of oil, sesame
- 1 tbsp. of minced garlic
- 1 tbsp. of peeled, grated ginger
- 1 chopped onion, yellow
- 3/4 pound of thinly sliced steak, top sirloin
- 1 tbsp. of soy sauce, low sodium
- 1 & 1/2 tbsp. of vinegar, red wine
- 1 tsp. of salt, kosher

Instructions:

Add the oil to large-sized frying pan on med. heat. Sauté the onions, garlic and ginger for two to three minutes. Add steak slices. Stir till cooked through, five minutes or so.

Add vinegar, soy sauce & salt. Stir till coated well. Toss in the avocado cubes and serve.

10 – Avocado Chickpea Salad

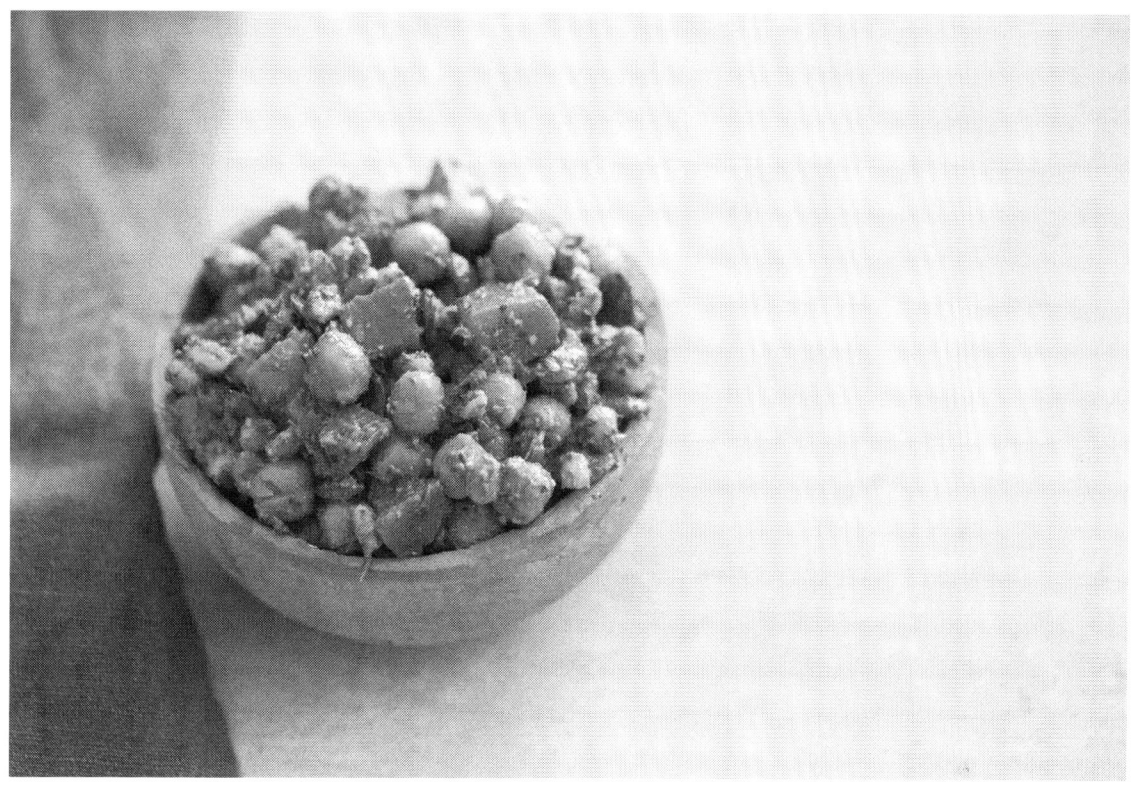

This salad is so tasty and it doesn't need dressing. The avocado moistens it and the salt gives it just enough flavor.

Makes 1 Serving

Cooking + Prep Time: 5-7 minutes

Ingredients:

- 1/2 cup of cooked chickpeas
- 1/3 small or medium avocado
- 1 & 3/4 ounce of tomatoes, grape
- 1 tsp. of hemp seeds
- 1/4 tsp. of salt, sea

Instructions:

Drain, then rinse chickpeas.

Chop grape tomatoes and avocado.

Mix all ingredients in large-sized bowl and serve.

11 – Chicken Cacciatore

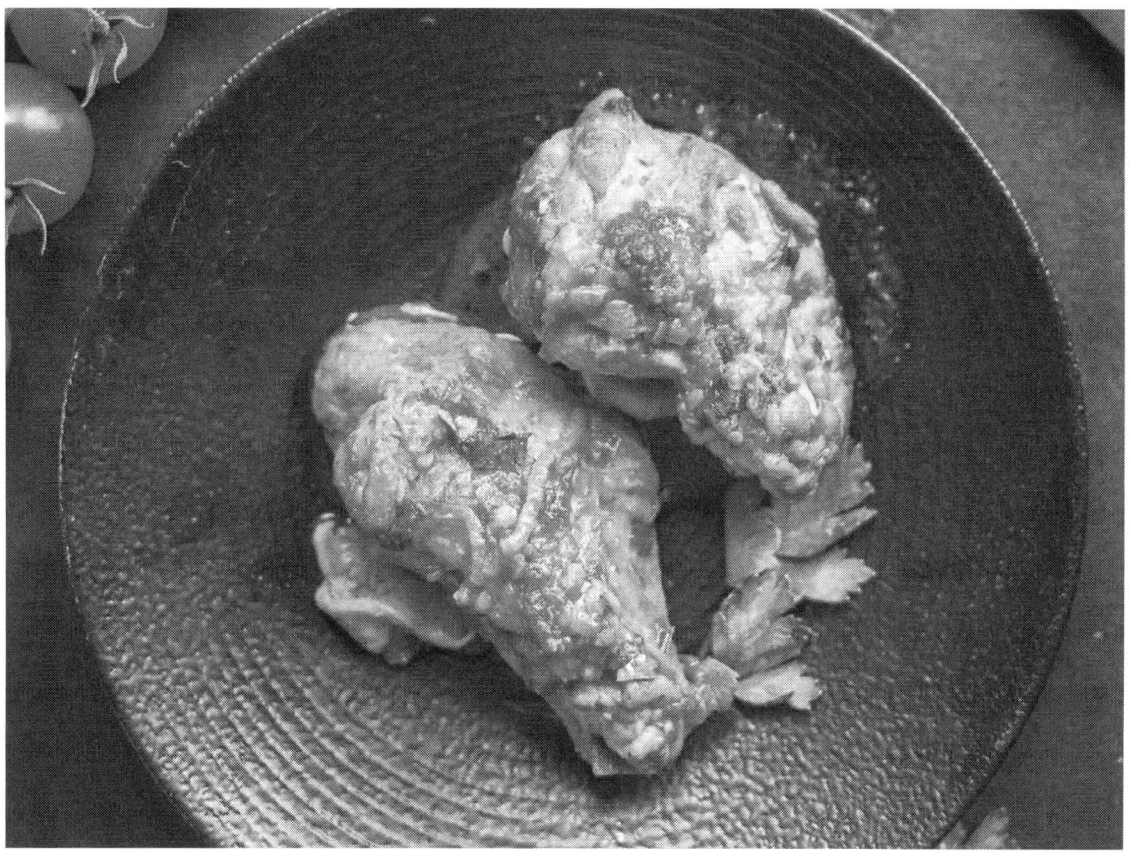

This is an easy dish to make, and it tastes great on couscous or zoodles. Serve a fresh side salad to make this a meal that everyone will love.

Makes various # of Servings

Cooking + Prep Time: 30 minutes

Ingredients:

- 1/4 cup of flour, almond
- 1 pound of chicken breast, skinless, boneless
- 2 tsp. of oil, olive
- 1 chopped onion, small
- 8 ounces of mushrooms, sliced
- 1 tsp. of rosemary, dried
- 1 x 14-ounce can of tomatoes, diced
- 1 cup of chicken broth, low sodium
- Salt, kosher, as desired
- Pepper, ground, as desired

Instructions:

Halve chicken breast lengthways. Coat with flour.

Heat 1 tsp. oil on med-high in large pan. Add chicken. Cook for five minutes per side. Remove the chicken breasts from the pan.

In same pan, add onions, mushrooms & rosemary & cook till they brown.

Add the tomatoes and broth. Allow to simmer for five minutes. Place chicken back in pan. Cook for five more minutes, till internal temp. reaches 165F. Serve.

12 – Chicken Tortilla Soup

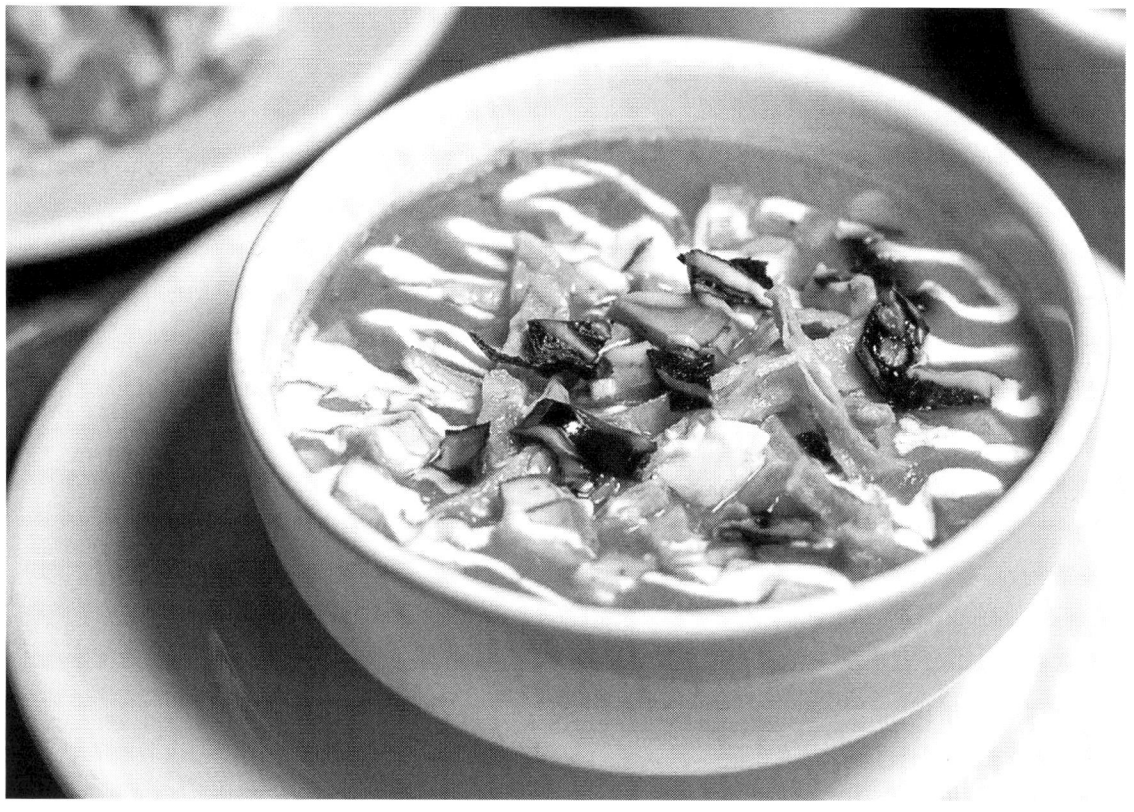

This soup can be made with chicken breasts or tenderloins. The slow cooker will do most of the cooking work for you.

Makes 8-10 Servings

Cooking + Prep Time: 25 minutes + 6 hours slow cooker time

Ingredients:

- 1 pound of tenderloins, chicken breast
- 1 tsp. of pepper, ground
- 1 tsp. of salt, kosher
- 2 cups of black bean salsa, prepared
- 2 tsp. of Mexican spice blend, mild
- 1 tsp. of cumin, ground
- 8 ounces of sliced queso blanco
- 4 cups of water, filtered
- 2 cups of corn, frozen
- Optional: 10 ounces of black beans
- 10 ounces of tomatoes, diced
- 4 & 1/2 ounces of green chilies, mild
- 2 tbsp. of chopped cilantro, fresh
- Optional: lime, fresh

Instructions:

Rinse the chicken tenderloins. Pat them dry. Season as desired and place in slow cooker.

Pour salsa atop chicken. Add the spices. Set slow cooker at four hours on the low setting.

Remove chicken when done fully through. Shred the meat and return to slow cooker.

Add water, extra beans, corn, tomatoes, cilantro and chilies. Let mixture cook for two more hours.

Squirt over top with lime juice and serve hot.

13 – Turkey Chili

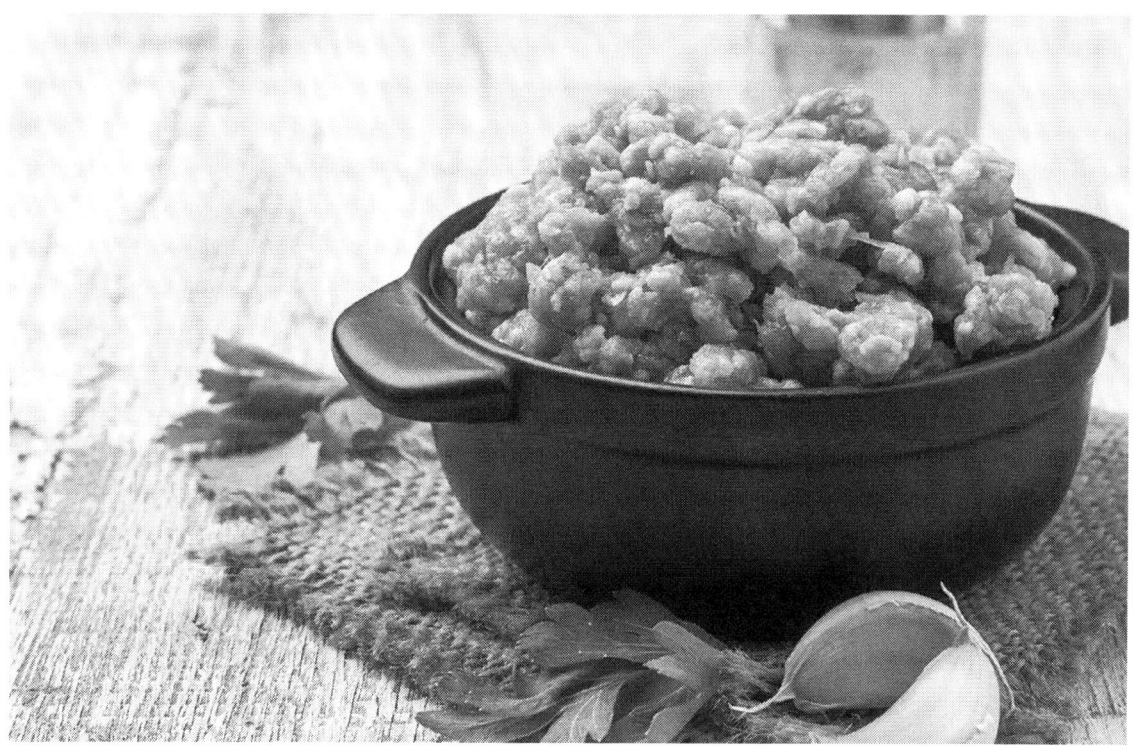

This turkey chili is so simple to make and you'll enjoy it quite often. Many of the ingredients are probably in your home pantry already.

Makes 6 Servings

Cooking + Prep Time: 1/2 hour

Ingredients:

- 2 tbsp. of oil, olive
- 1 pound of ground turkey, lean
- 1 chopped onion, medium
- 1 & 1/2 tsp. of cumin, ground
- 1 & 1/2 tbsp. of chili powder
- 1 x 28-ounce can of tomatoes, crushed
- 1 cup of chicken broth, low sodium
- 1 can of rinsed, drained kidney beans
- Salt, kosher, as desired
- Pepper, ground, as desired

Instructions:

Heat the oil in your Instant Pot. Add onion and sauté till softened.

Add turkey and spices. Sauté till turkey has browned.

Stir in broth and tomatoes. Close the lid. Cook on high setting for 8-10 minutes.

When done, release the valve. Add and stir in the beans and serve.

14 – Sausage & Summer Beans

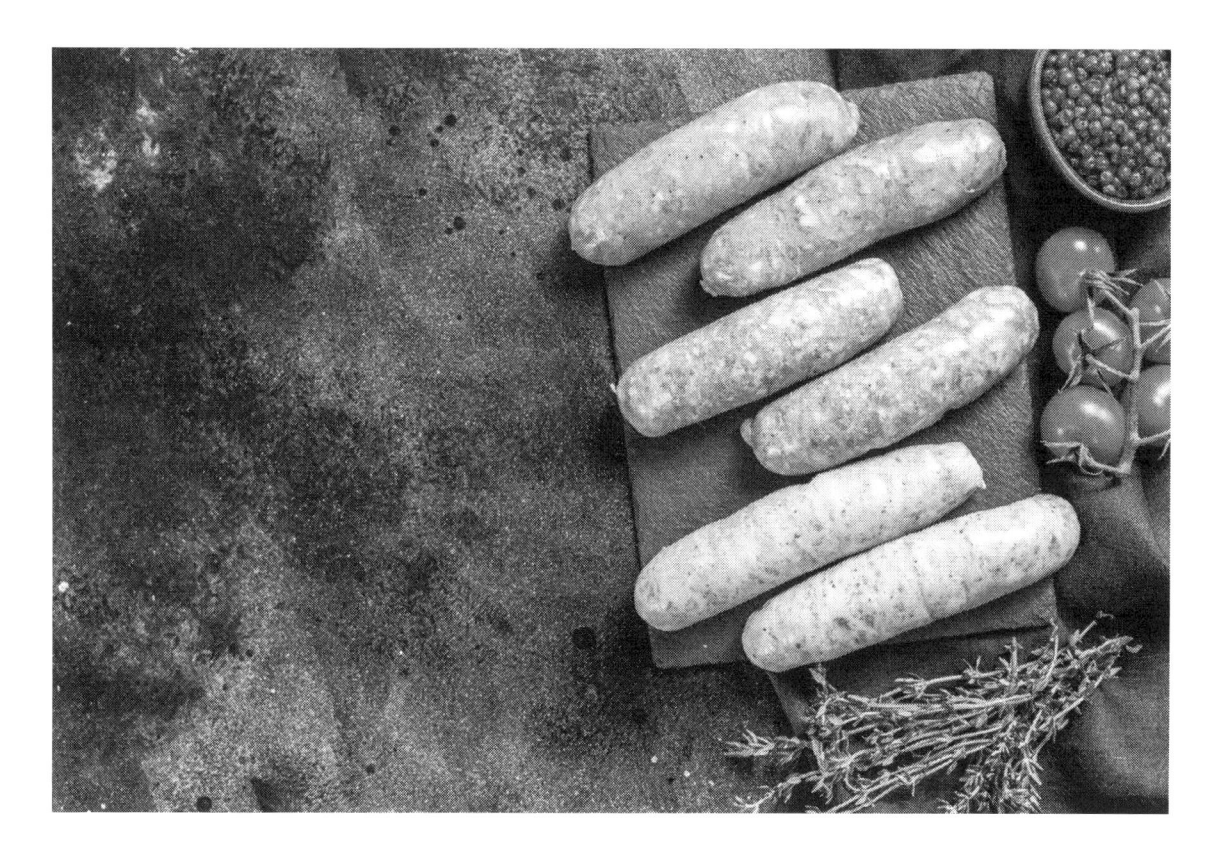

This tasty recipe is the post-bariatric surgery equivalent of BBQ beans. These are spicy and savory, but not overly so, and they blend well with other foods served with them.

Makes 6 Servings

Cooking + Prep Time: 15 minutes + 8 hours slow cooker time

Ingredients:

- 8 ounces of diced sausage, Andouille
- 1 chopped onion, yellow
- 2 de-seeded, diced tomatoes
- 3 minced garlic cloves
- 1 pound of dry beans, Great Northern
- 2 tsp. of spice blend, Cajun
- 1/2 tsp. of salt, kosher
- 1 tsp. of paprika, smoked
- 1 diced pepper, jalapeno
- 4 cups of chicken broth, low sodium
- 2 cups of water, filtered

Instructions:

Use non-stick spray on a large skillet. Set on med. heat & let it heat up.

Add the sausage. Cook till one side is browned. Add tomatoes and onions. Cook two minutes more. Add garlic and cook for one minute more.

Empty skillet contents into slow cooker. Top with the beans, peppers, broth, spices & water. Combine well.

Set slow cooker on the low setting. Let mixture cook for eight hours, till beans have completed cooking and liquid has thickened. Serve.

15 – Rosemary Lemon Chicken

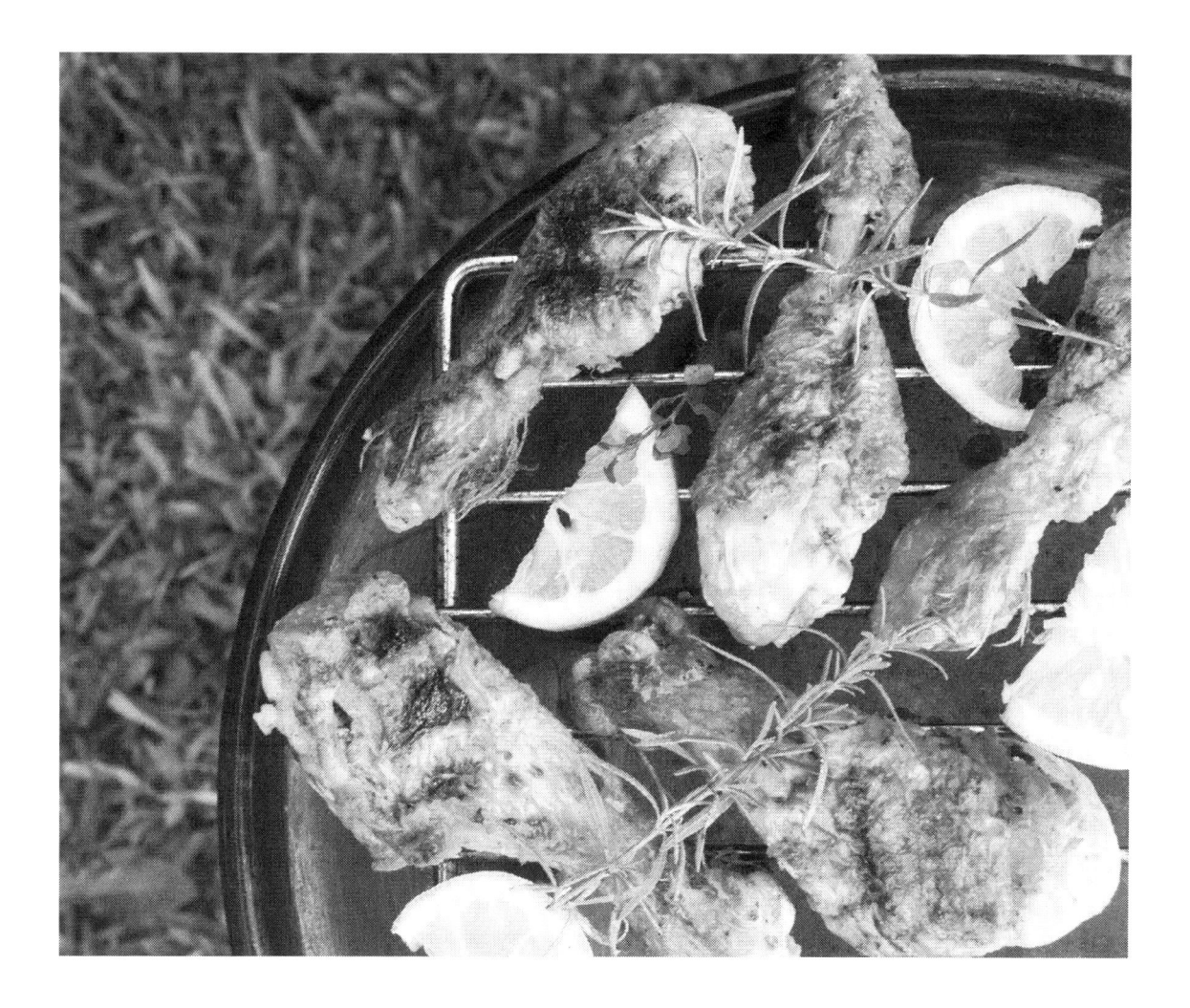

This chicken recipe is made in a sheet pan, so it's a perfect family meal. It's designed for post-bariatric surgery, but the taste is one that everyone will enjoy.

Makes 3-4 Servings

Cooking + Prep Time: 50 minutes

Ingredients:

- 1/4 cup of oil, olive
- 1 lemon, sliced
- 1 lemon, juiced
- 1 tbsp. of rosemary, dried
- 1 tsp. of garlic, minced
- 1/2 tsp. of salt, kosher
- 1/4 tsp. of pepper, ground
- 1 & 1/2 pounds of drumsticks, chicken
- 1 diced sweet potato, medium
- 3 round-cut carrots, medium

Instructions:

Heat the oven to 425F.

In small sized bowl, mix oil, lemon juice, garlic, rosemary, kosher salt & ground pepper together.

In larger bowl, add chicken, sweet potatoes and carrots. Toss with dressing prepared above.

Place mixture in one layer in casserole dish. Top with the sliced lemon. Cook in 425F oven for 30-35 minutes, till internal temp has reached 165F. Serve.

16 – Couscous & Veggies

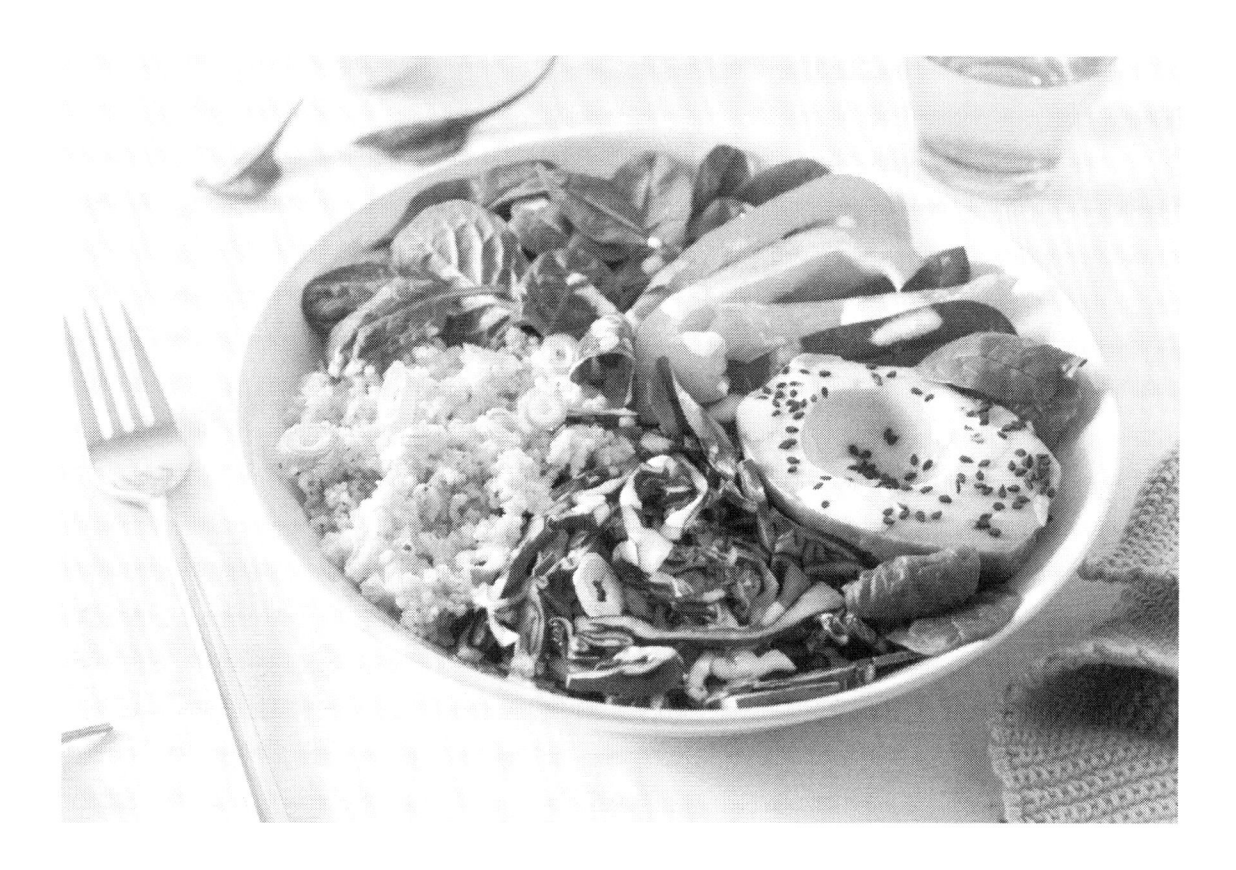

This dish is easy to make with boxed, cooked couscous, and roasted vegetables. You can roast garlic with the vegetables, then dice it and mix it with veggies, too, for added flavor.

Makes 8 Servings

Cooking + Prep Time: 1/2 hour

Ingredients:

- 10 ounces box couscous, store bought
- Butter or oil for preparing couscous
- 2 to 3 cups of vegetables, roasted
- Salt, kosher, as desired
- Pepper, ground, as desired
- Optional: Parmesan cheese, freshly shaved
- 1 pound of small-diced chicken breast, pre-cooked

Instructions:

Cook the couscous using instructions on box.

Add the roasted veggies to the pot while the couscous is still nice and hot. Add chicken, too.

Toss with your preferred seasonings. Top with grated Parmesan cheese, as desired, and serve.

17 – Squash Soup

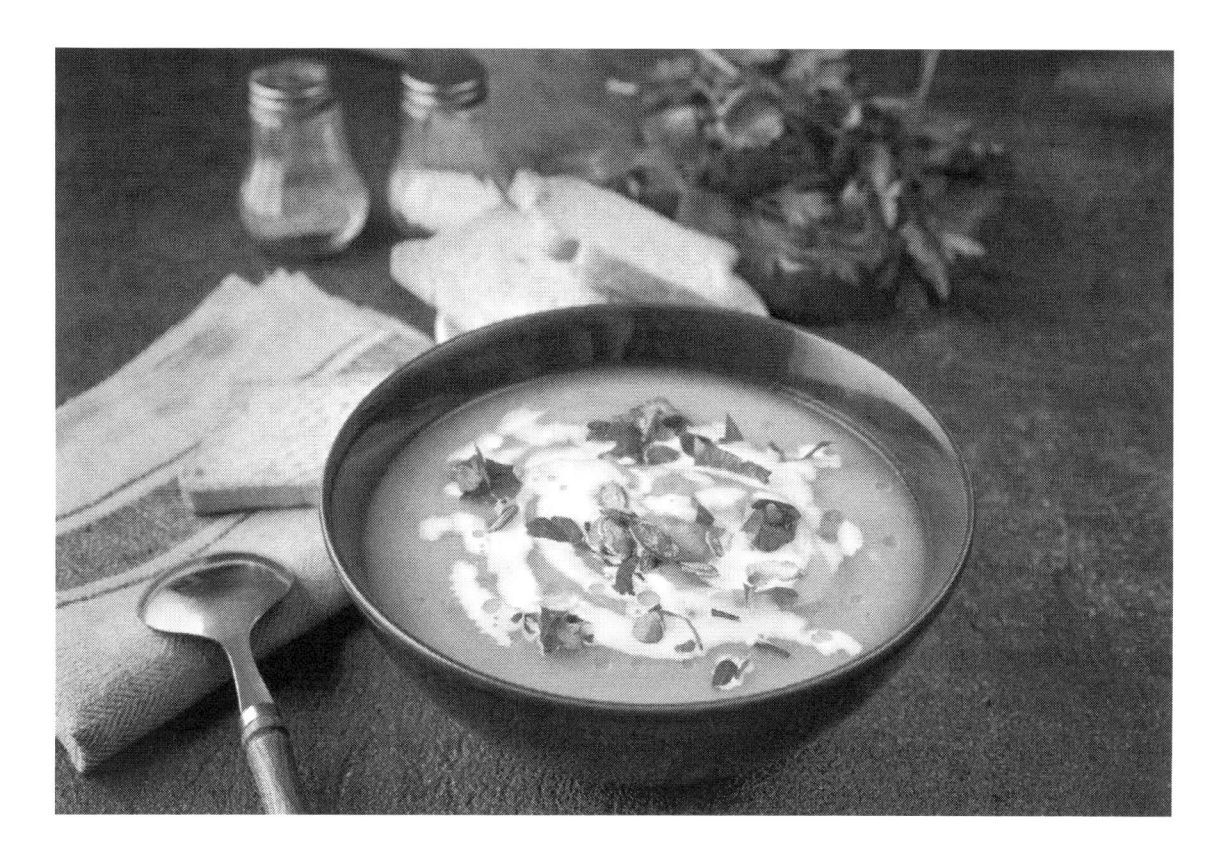

Butternut squash is a high-protein ingredient that makes a wonderful comfort food soup, especially during the winter. It is suitable for nearly any post-bariatric stage.

Makes 2 Servings

Cooking + Prep Time: 35 minutes

Ingredients:

- 1/2 pound of squash, butternut
- 1 tsp. of oil, olive
- 1/2 diced onion, medium
- 32 ounces soup base, almond milk
- 1 tsp. of minced, ginger
- 1 tsp. of garlic powder
- Salt, kosher, as desired
- Pepper, ground, as desired
- 2 scoops of protein powder, unflavored

Instructions:

Sauté the onion in oil in pan on med. heat till it becomes translucent. Add garlic and ginger. Sauté for a minute more.

Add soup base, squash & seasonings. Bring to boil. Allow to simmer for 12-15 minutes, till squash becomes soft.

Puree soup in blender. When temperature is lower than 140F, add the protein powder and mix well before serving.

18 – Turkey Cabbage Rolls

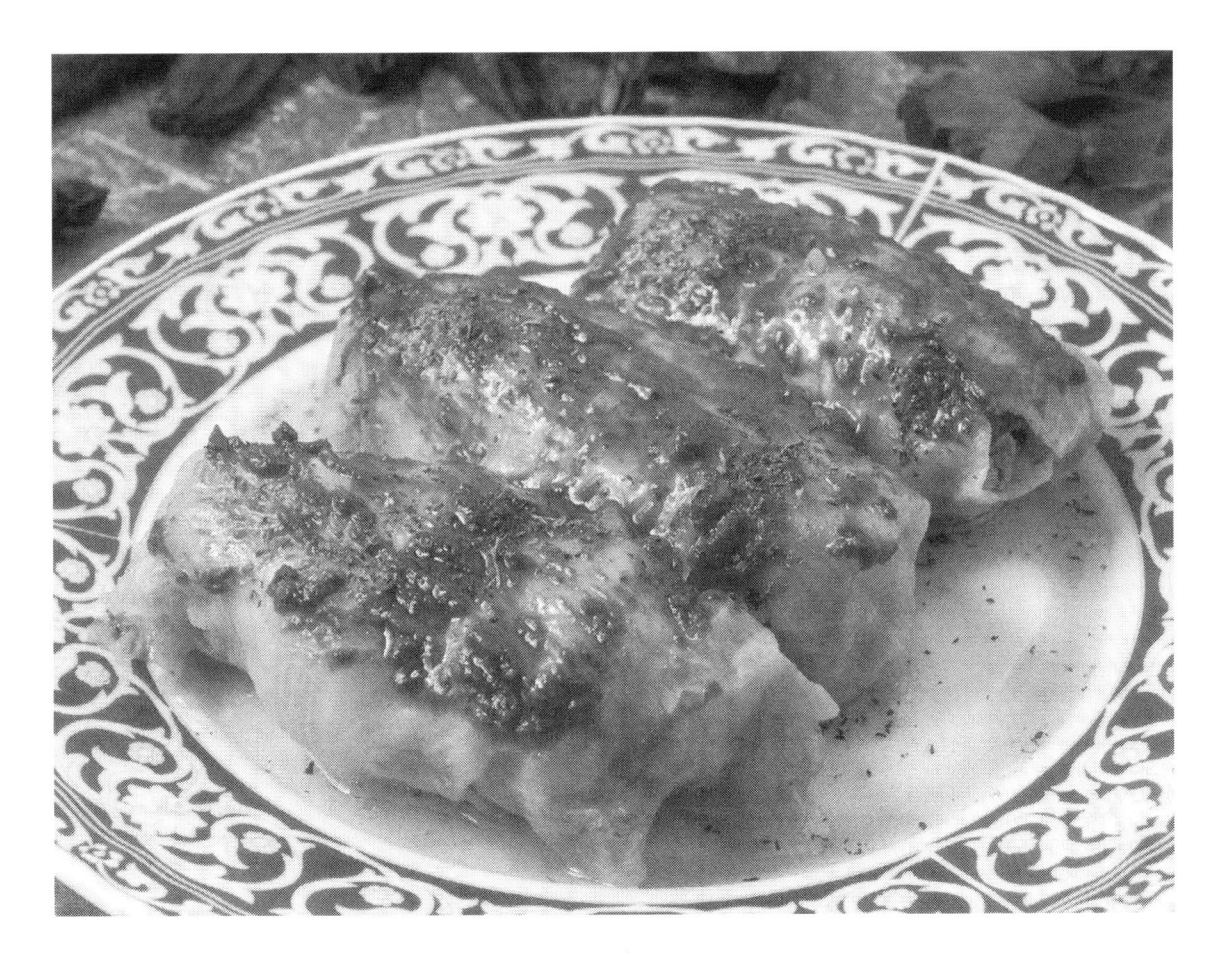

These cabbage rolls certainly are a traditional comfort food. This recipe offers you a soothing meal for those cold winter days.

Makes 12 Servings

Cooking + Prep Time: 55 minutes

Ingredients:

- 12 leaves of cabbage
- 1 diced medium onion, yellow
- 1 pound of ground turkey, lean
- 1 cup of cauliflower rice
- 1/4 tsp. of salt, kosher
- 1/4 tsp. of pepper, ground
- 2 tbsp. of paprika, smoked
- 1/2 tsp. of seasoning blend, Italian
- 2 tbsp. of Worcestershire sauce, low sodium
- 1 x 10-ounce can of tomatoes, whole, no salt added
- 1/2 tsp. of onion powder
- 1/2 tsp. of garlic powder
- 1 tsp. of sweetener, zero calorie

Instructions:

Preheat oven to 350F.

Bring large pot with water to full boil. Place metal colander over the pot. Drop leaves of cabbage in colander and let them steam till somewhat softened. Place in bowl. Set them aside.

Use non-stick spray on a skillet. Set on med. heat and let it get hot.

Sauté the onions in skillet for one to two minutes, till they soften. Add the turkey and allow to completely brown.

Add spices and seasonings + 1 tbsp. Worcestershire sauce. Stir and blend well. Add the cauliflower rice. Let mixture cook another two to three minutes.

In food processor, pulse the tomatoes and liquid till mixture is fully liquified. Add remainder of spices and Worcestershire sauce. Pulse mixture again.

For roll assembly, lay steamed cabbage leaf on clean work surface. Spoon on 2 oz. of meat mixture. Fold the long ends in. Roll lengthwise, like a burrito. Place in baking dish.

Repeat step 7 with remainder of cabbage and fillings. Pour the tomato sauce over the top. Heat in 350F oven and serve.

19 – Tofu Salad

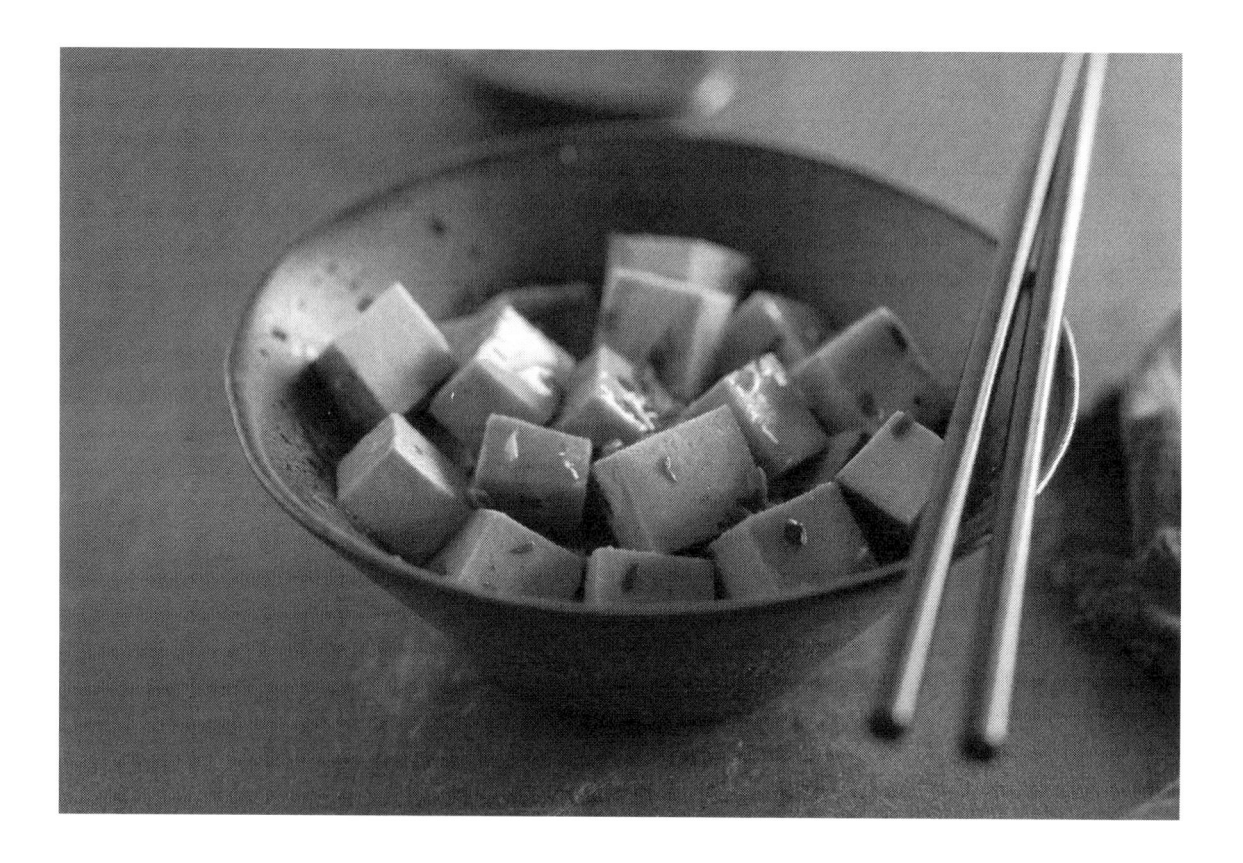

Sometimes, dishes without meat are a nice break after bariatric surgery. This salad is made with tofu, and it's satisfying yet simple.

Makes 4 Servings

Cooking + Prep Time: 55 minutes

Ingredients:

- 1 pound of tofu, extra firm
- 1/4 cup peanut sauce, Thai
- 2 tsp. of oil, sesame
- 2 cups of coleslaw mix
- 1/3 cup of green onions, chopped
- Vinegar, apple cider

Instructions:

Remove the tofu from its package. Press well, removing liquid.

Cut tofu into cubes. Place them in medium bowl. Toss with peanut sauce. Place in the refrigerator for 18-20 minutes. Once tofu has marinated, remove it from the refrigerator.

Heat oil in frying pan. Add tofu. Stir-fry for 8-10 minutes, till all sides have turned golden brown in color. Remove pan from heat.

Transfer to large bowl. Add 1/2 cup coleslaw mixture and green onions to garnish. Drizzle vinegar over the top. Serve.

20 – Apple & Pork Stew

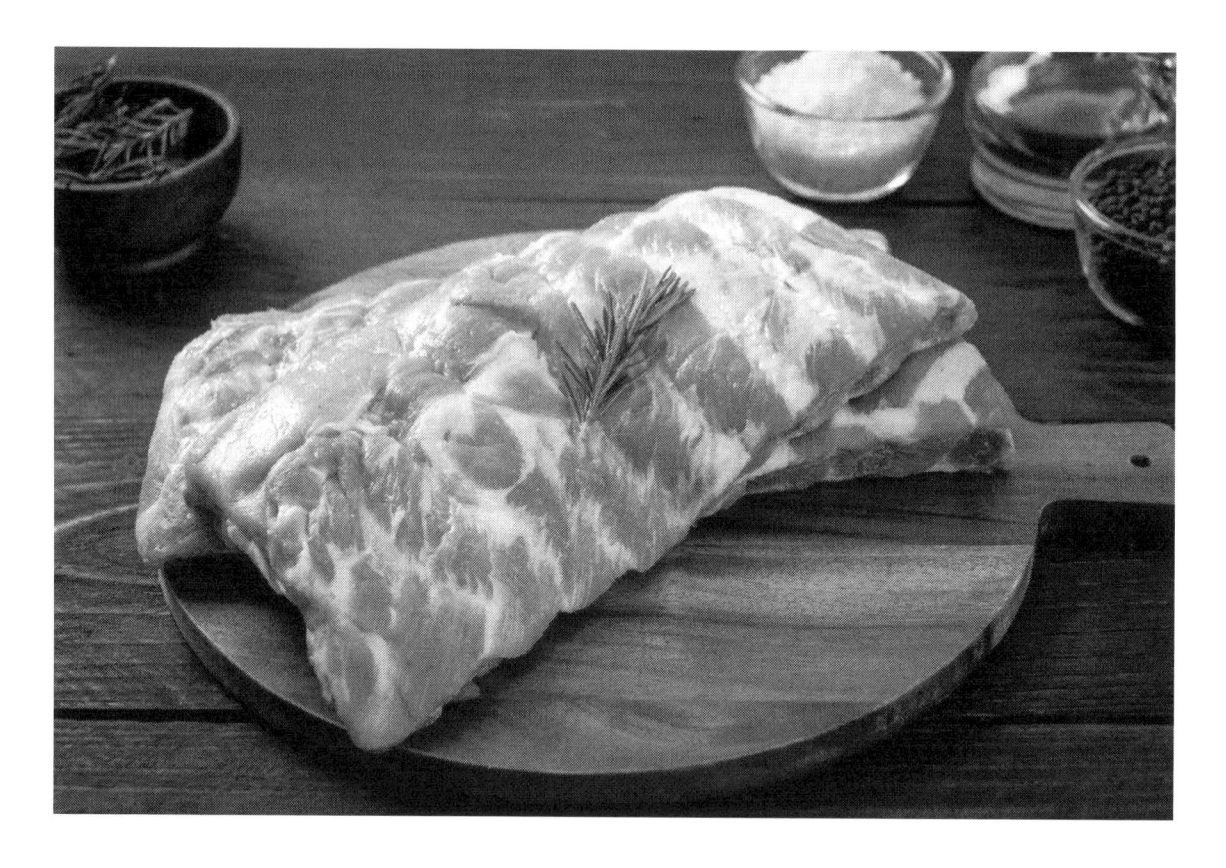

This recipe contains a variety of spices, but you don't need them all. Choose from among your favorites and tailor the dish to yourself and your family.

Makes 8 Servings

Cooking + Prep Time: 20 minutes + 5 hours slow cooker time

Ingredients:

- 3 diced bacon slices
- 2 pounds of cubed country ribs, pork
- 1 sliver-cut medium onion, yellow
- 1 tsp. of salt, kosher
- 1/2 tsp. of pepper, ground
- 1 tsp. of sage, dried
- 1 tsp. of minced garlic, fresh
- 1 tsp. of ginger, ground
- 1 tsp. of mustard, Dijon
- 1 tsp. of chopped basil leaves
- 1/2 tsp. of nutmeg, ground
- 4 cups of chicken broth, low sodium
- 1 cup of cider, hard
- 1/4 cup of vinegar, apple cider
- 3 cups of diced butternut squash or sweet potato
- 3 peeled, then cored & sliced Honeycrisp apples, medium

Instructions:

In stovetop setting of slow cooker, set to med. Add pieces of bacon. Fry, rendering the fat. Remove bacon and reserve for later use. Turn slow cooker to high. Add the ribs and sear them on each side. Remove ribs.

In small mixing bowl, mix herbs & spices together loosely. Add mustard, onions and spices to slow cooker. Stir till all remaining fat from bacon has been incorporated. Add ribs back into slow cooker.

Add squash or sweet potatoes, then broth and cider. Set slow cooker on the low setting for four hours.

Add the apple slices. Cook for another hour. Serve hot.

21 – Stuffed Apple Pork Chops

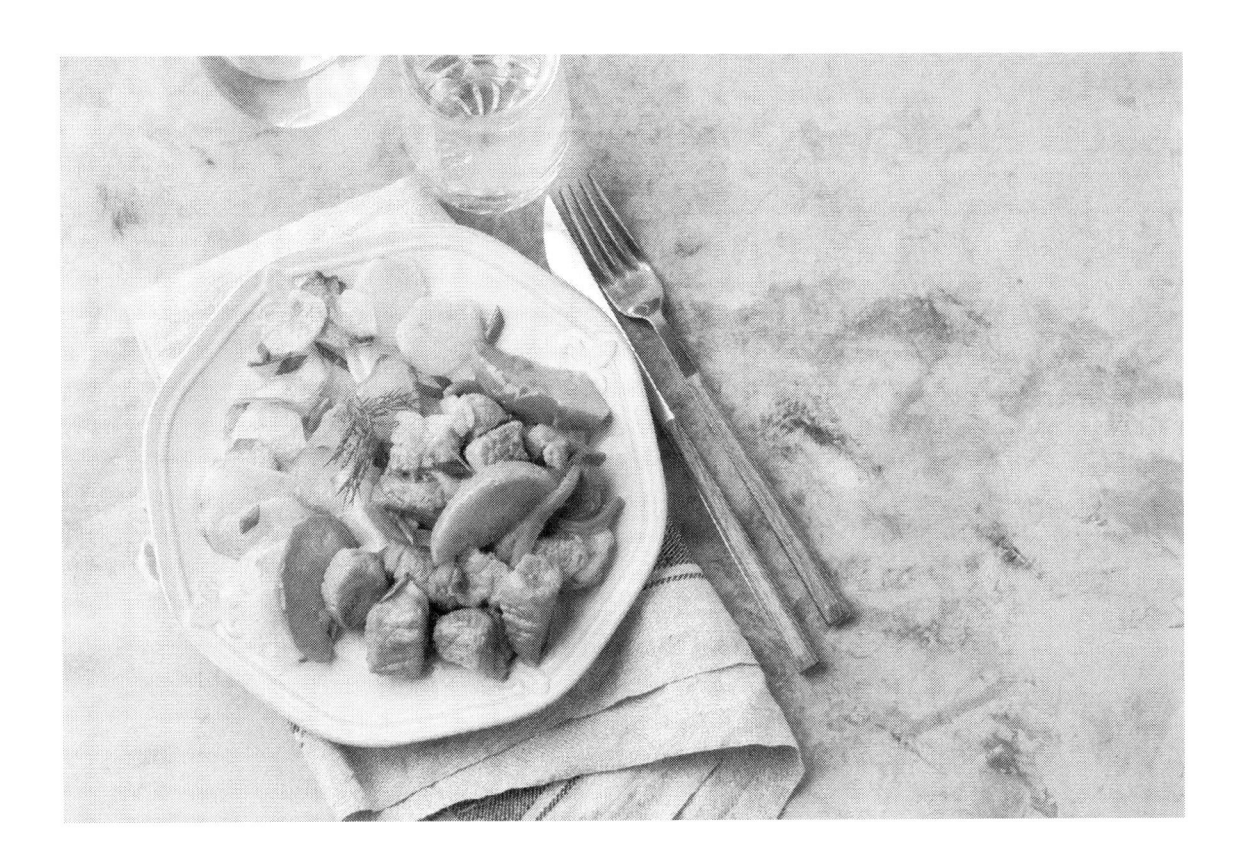

These pork chops are a wonderful blend of sweet and savory. The tastes will definitely satisfy you, your family, and guests.

Makes 4 Servings

Cooking + Prep Time: 50 minutes

Ingredients:

- 4 pork chops, thick-cut, bone-in

For the stuffing

- 1 tbsp. butter, unsalted
- 1/2 chopped onion, sweet
- 1 tsp. of sage, dried
- 1/2 chopped apple, medium
- 1/4 cup of dried cranberries
- Salt, kosher, as desired
- Pepper, ground, as desired

Instructions:

Preheat oven to 375F.

Heat unsalted butter in a skillet on med. heat. Add the onions. Sauté for five minutes or so, till slightly browned and softened.

Add cranberries, sage and apples. Sauté for 8-10 minutes more, till apples soften. Season as desired. Remove pan from heat. Set it aside.

Cut slits in pork chops, creating pockets. Fill pockets with apple stuffing prepared above.

Place pork chops in a baking dish. Place in 375F oven for 1/2 hour, till the internal temperature has reached 145F. Serve.

22 – Chicken Salad with Pecans & Apples

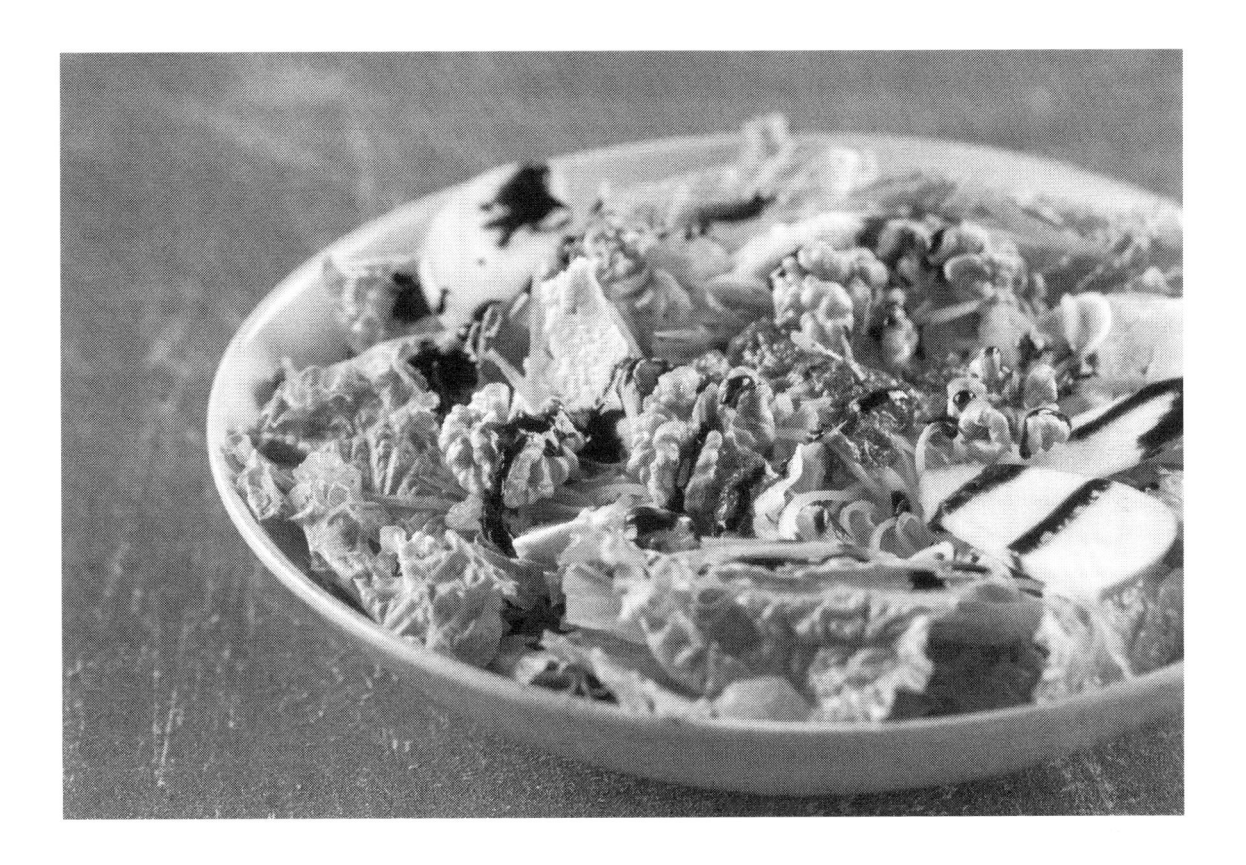

This wonderful dish has chicken for the savory taste, then pecans and apples for crunch and extra flavor. It's like a meal in a dish.

Makes 1-2 Servings

Cooking + Prep Time: 5-7 minutes

Ingredients:

- 4 ounces of shredded or diced chicken breast, cooked
- 2 tbsp. of minced or diced onion, yellow
- 1/2 of 1 apple, diced, sweet
- 2 tbsp. of pecan pieces, crushed
- 2 tsp. of mustard, Dijon
- 1/4 tsp. of garlic powder
- 1 tbsp. of mayonnaise, low fat
- Salt, kosher, as desired
- Pepper, ground, as desired

Instructions:

Combine all the ingredients in bowl. Mix well. Place in refrigerator till ready to serve.

23 – Cauliflower Bake

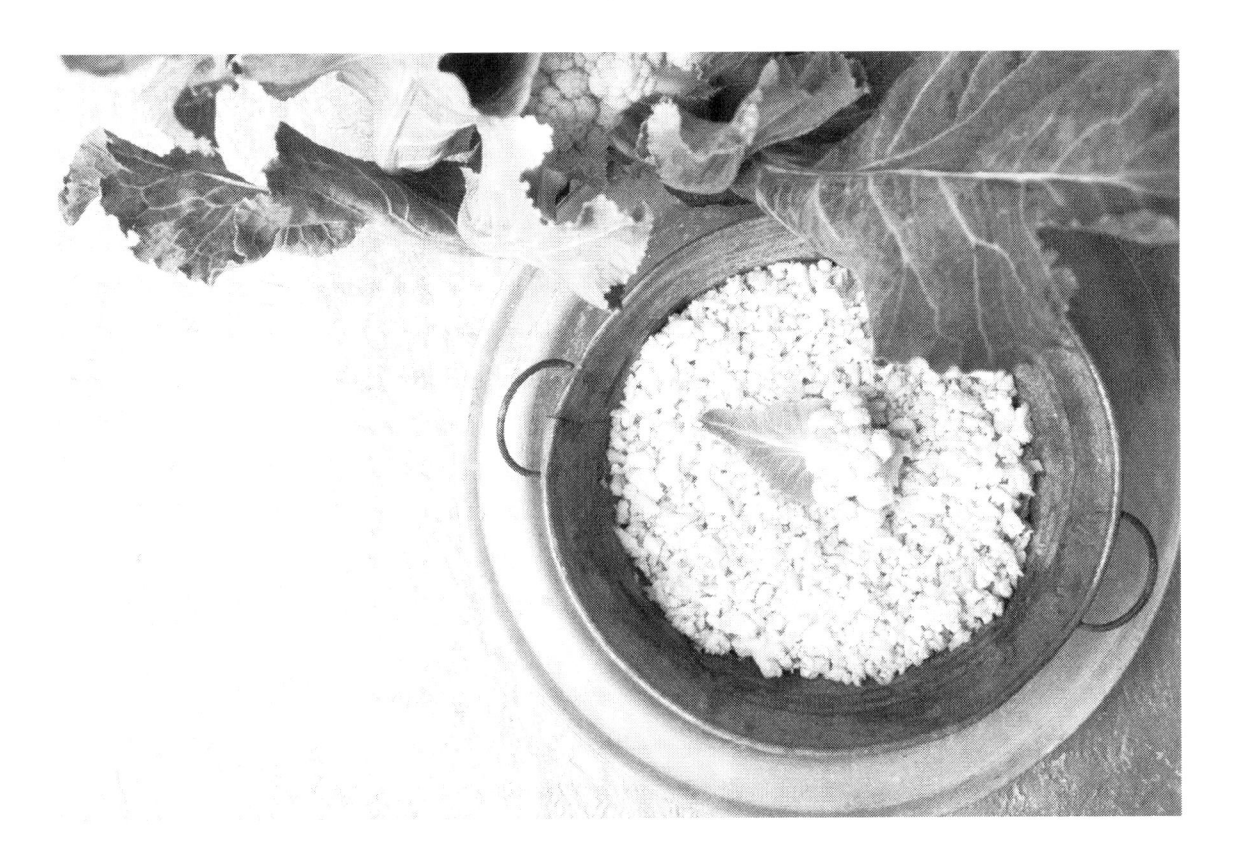

This cauliflower bake is very popular after bariatric surgery. Making it in a mug is so easy since they're one serving and quick to prepare.

Makes 1 Serving

Cooking + Prep Time: 5-7 minutes

Ingredients:

- 1/3 cup of cauliflower rice
- 1/4 cup of tomato sauce, no sugar added
- 1/2 cup of cheese, ricotta
- Optional: 1 tbsp. of cheese, mozzarella

Instructions:

Add 1/3 cup cauliflower rice to mug. Top with 1/4 cup marinara sauce & 1/2 cup ricotta. Mix them together well.

Place mug in the microwave. Cook for three to four minutes on the high setting. Remove the mug. Add a tbsp. of mozzarella cheese, as desired. Place mug back into microwave for 20 more seconds. Allow to cool a bit and serve.

24 – Steak Fajitas

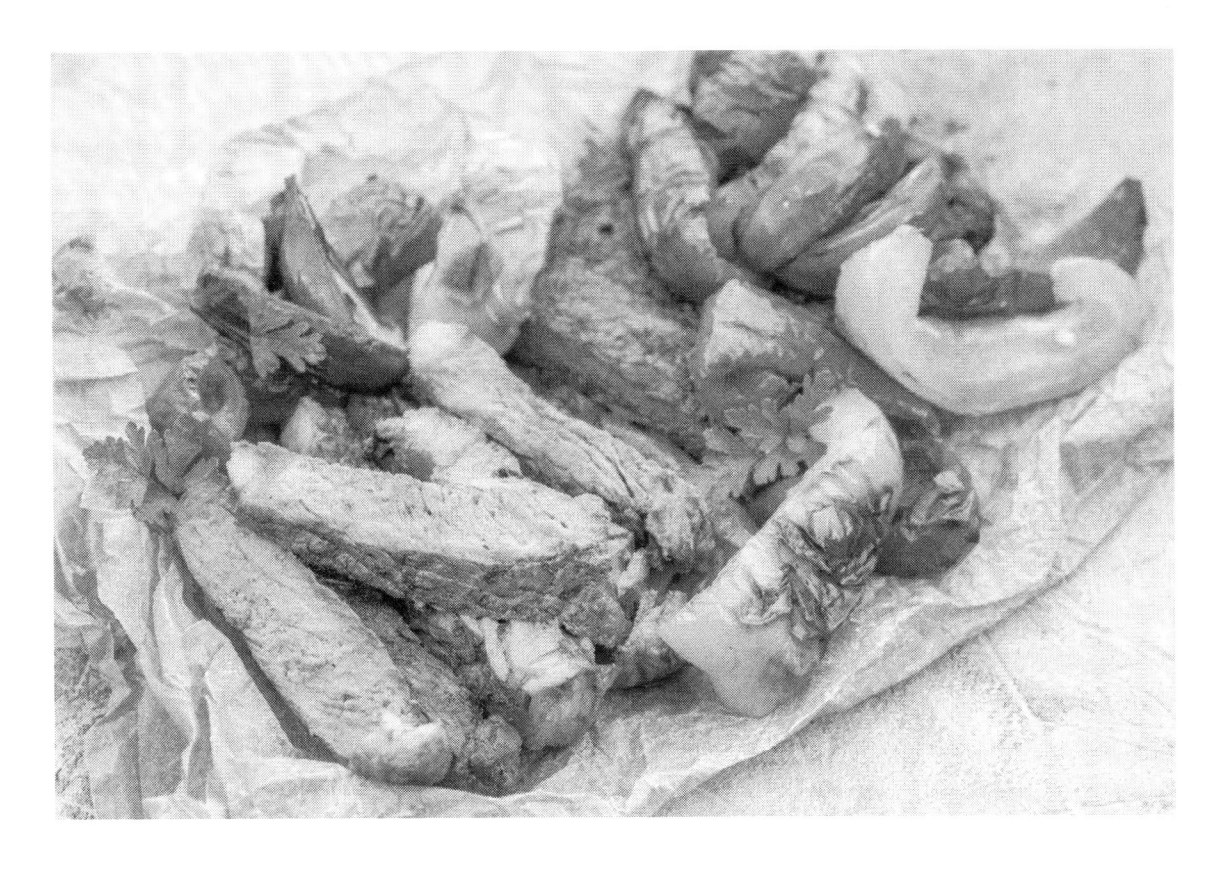

This is an easy recipe – you don't have to do lots of prep work, and it doesn't require numerous pots & pans. It's ready quickly and it disappears fast!

Makes 4 Servings

Cooking + Prep Time: 45 minutes

Ingredients:

- 1 tbsp. of oil, olive
- 1 strip-cut medium onion, yellow
- 1 seeded, strip-cut bell pepper, red
- 1 seeded, strip-cut bell pepper, yellow
- 2 tsp. of minced garlic
- 1/2 pound of steak, thin cut in strips
- Salt, kosher as desired
- Pepper, ground as desired
- 1 tsp. of cumin, ground
- 1 tsp. of coriander, ground
- 1 tsp. of chili pepper
- 1 pinch pepper, cayenne
- 4 cups of cauliflower rice, frozen
- 2 tbsp. of tomato paste, no salt added
- 1/3 cup of water, filtered

Instructions:

Place skillet on med. heat. Let it heat up. Add the oil.

Sauté the garlic, onions and peppers till they soften, five to seven minutes.

As veggies sauté, place strips of steak in medium bowl. Toss with 1/2 of each spice type and 1/2 kosher salt & ground pepper.

Add the steak to skillet. Sauté till it browns.

Add the cauliflower rice. Combine well and cook till it thaws. Add tomato paste, remainder of spices and filtered water, as needed.

Reduce the heat level to med-low. Cover skillet. Let mixture cook while stirring frequently for 10 to 15 minutes.

Season as desired. Serve.

25 – Chicken Lentil Soup

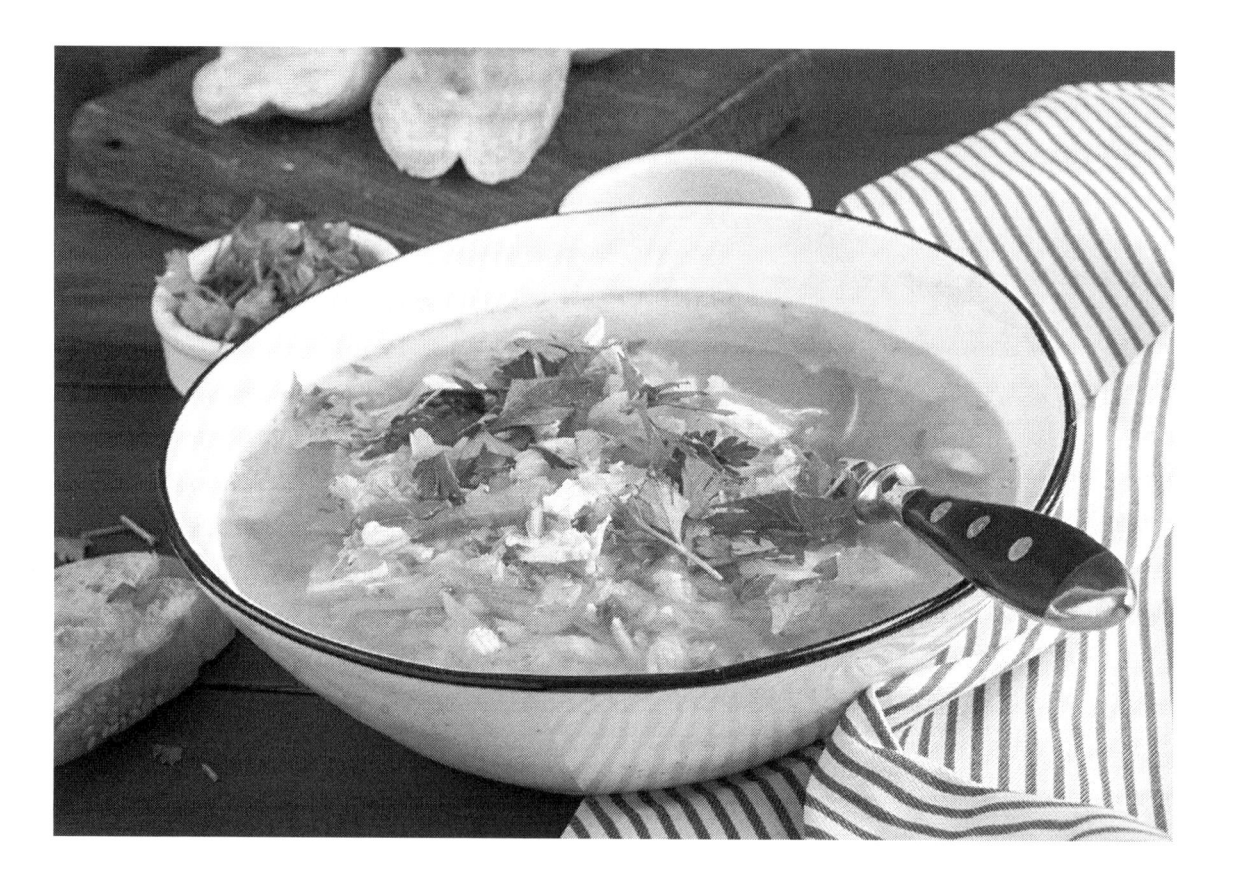

This soup can be made without chicken, but the protein is helpful if you've had bariatric surgery. The chicken and lentils go together so well.

Makes Various # of Servings

Cooking + Prep Time: 20 minutes

Ingredients:

- 1 tbsp. of oil, olive
- 1 peeled, diced medium onion, yellow
- 2 diced carrots, medium
- 1 tbsp. of garlic, minced
- 4 cups of stock, chicken, low sodium
- 1 cup of rinsed lentils, red
- 1 pound of chicken breast meat
- 1 tsp. of curry powder
- 2 tsp. of cumin, ground
- Salt, sea as desired
- Pepper, cracked, as desired

Instructions:

Press the "Sauté" setting on your Instant Pot. Add oil. After it heats, add the onion. Sauté for five minutes. Add garlic and carrots. Sauté for a minute more.

Add stock, chicken, spices and lentils. Press "Manual" setting. Set to pressure cook for 10 minutes. Once it's done, allow pressure to go down and then remove lid carefully.

Remove the chicken. Shred meat. Place meat back in Instant Pot. Stir well. Season as desired. Serve.

26 – Flounder & Roasted Vegetables

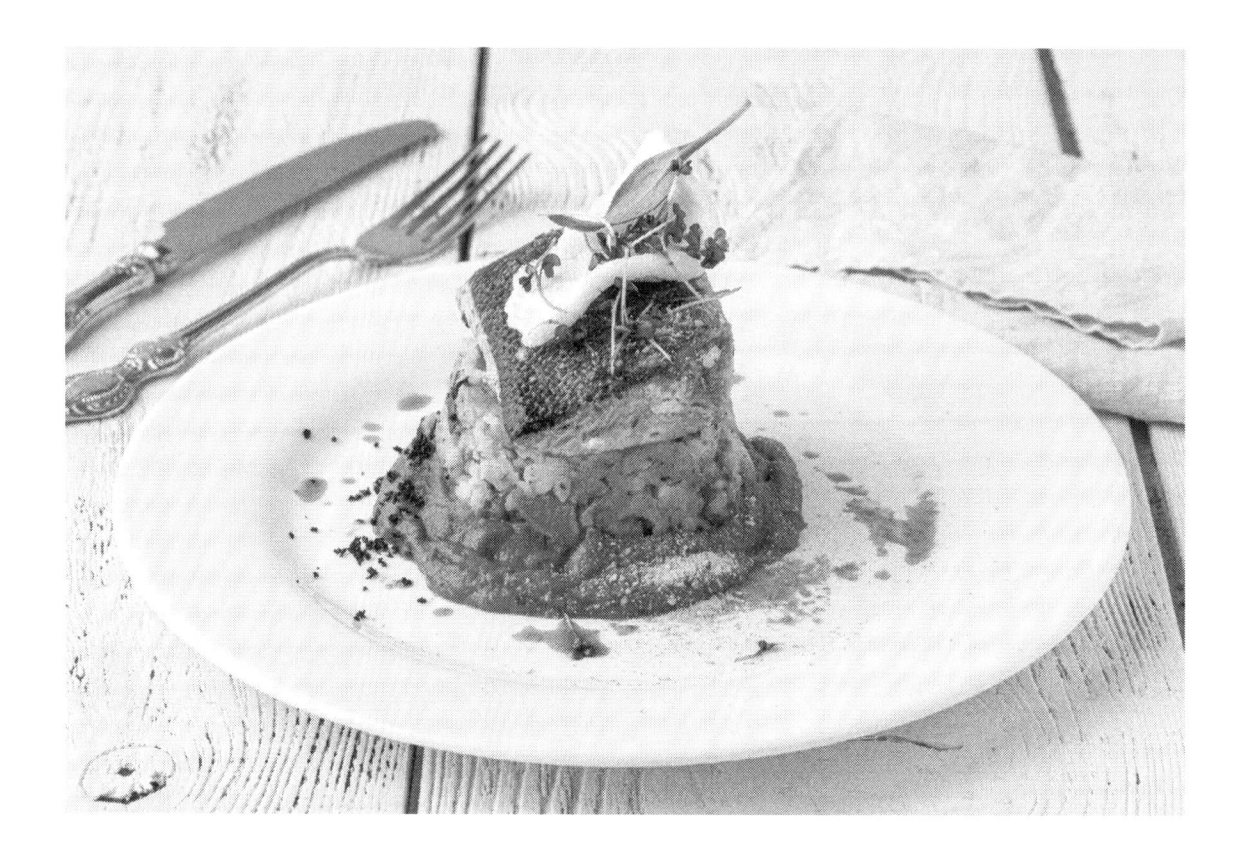

My family members are not fish "nuts", but I had the fish and needed to use it, so I prepared this dish for us. What a pleasing surprise! The vegetables have flavors and textures that complement the fish quite nicely.

Makes 4 servings with fish & vegetables

Cooking plus Prep Time: 45 minutes

Ingredients:

- 1 pound of flounder, frozen/thawed or fresh
- 1/2 cup of Parmesan cheese, grated, low-fat
- 1/4 tsp. salt, kosher
- 1/4 tsp. pepper, ground
- 1 strip-cut large bell pepper, yellow
- 1 cup of tomatoes, cherry
- 1/4 cup of hazelnuts, chopped

Instructions:

Preheat the oven to 400 degrees F.

Place the fish on cookie sheet. Coat each side using grated Parmesan. Season as desired. Add some chopped nuts to tops of fillets.

Add tomatoes and bell peppers to pan and surround fish with them.

Roast in 400F oven for 18-22 minutes, till vegetables have roasted and fish becomes flaky. Serve promptly.

27 – French Onion & Leek Soup

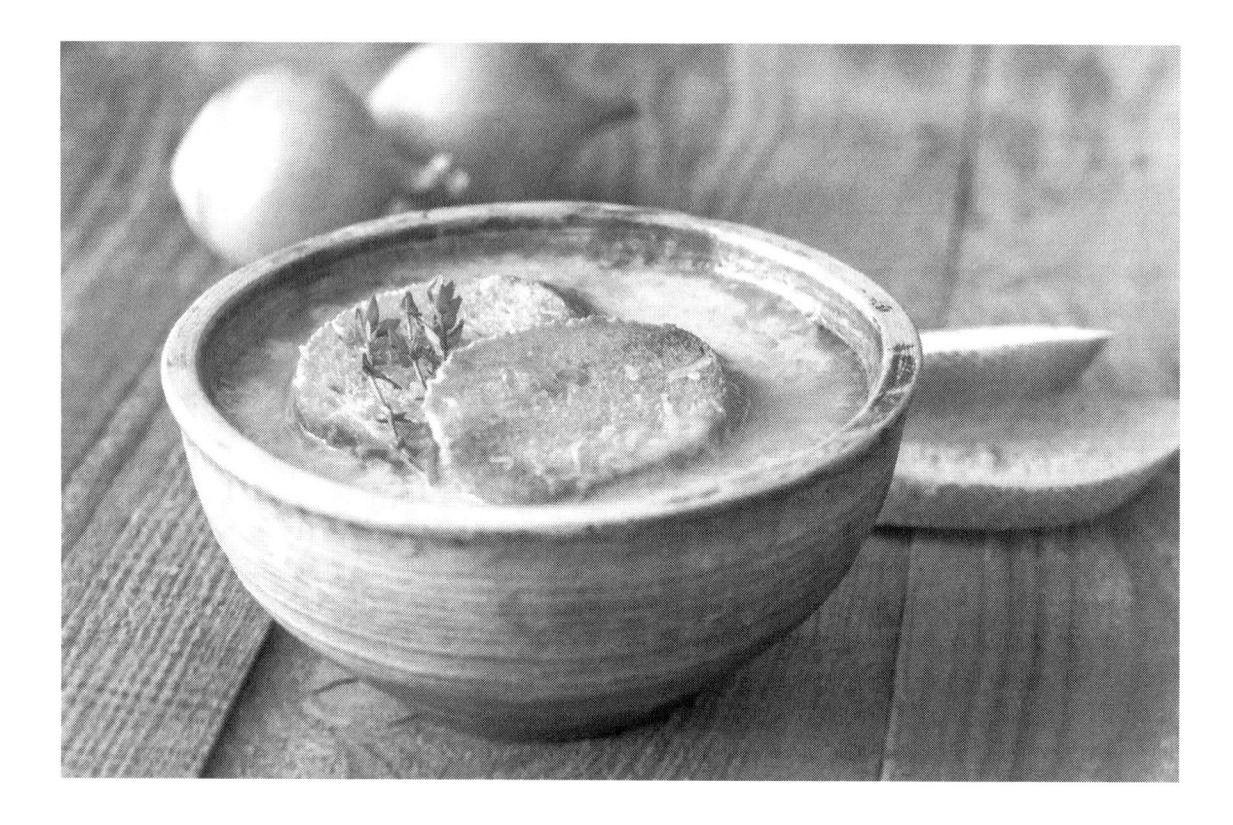

The best tip for the great onion soup is caramelizing your onions. Cook them on low to medium heat when you caramelize them, so they don't have any burned flavor.

Makes 4 Servings

Cooking + Prep Time: 1 hour

Ingredients:

- 1 tbsp. of oil, olive
- 2 peeled, thin-sliced medium onions, yellow or red
- 1 cleaned, thin-sliced leek, fresh
- 3 & 1/2 cups beef stock, low sodium
- 2 minced garlic cloves
- 1/4 tsp. of thyme, fresh
- 1 tsp. Worcestershire sauce, reduced sodium
- Salt, kosher, as desired
- Pepper, ground, as desired
- 1 tbsp. of cheese, shredded, low-fat

Instructions:

In medium-sized pot, add oil and bring to heat on med-low. Sauté the leeks and onions till tender. Don't let the leeks or onions burn at all.

Add garlic and stir.

Add stock. Bring mixture to a boil.

Reduce the heat to low. Cover pot. Simmer for 1/2 hour.

Turn heat off. Blend soup in food processor.

Garnish with shredded cheese. Season as desired and serve.

28 – Turkey Taco Casserole

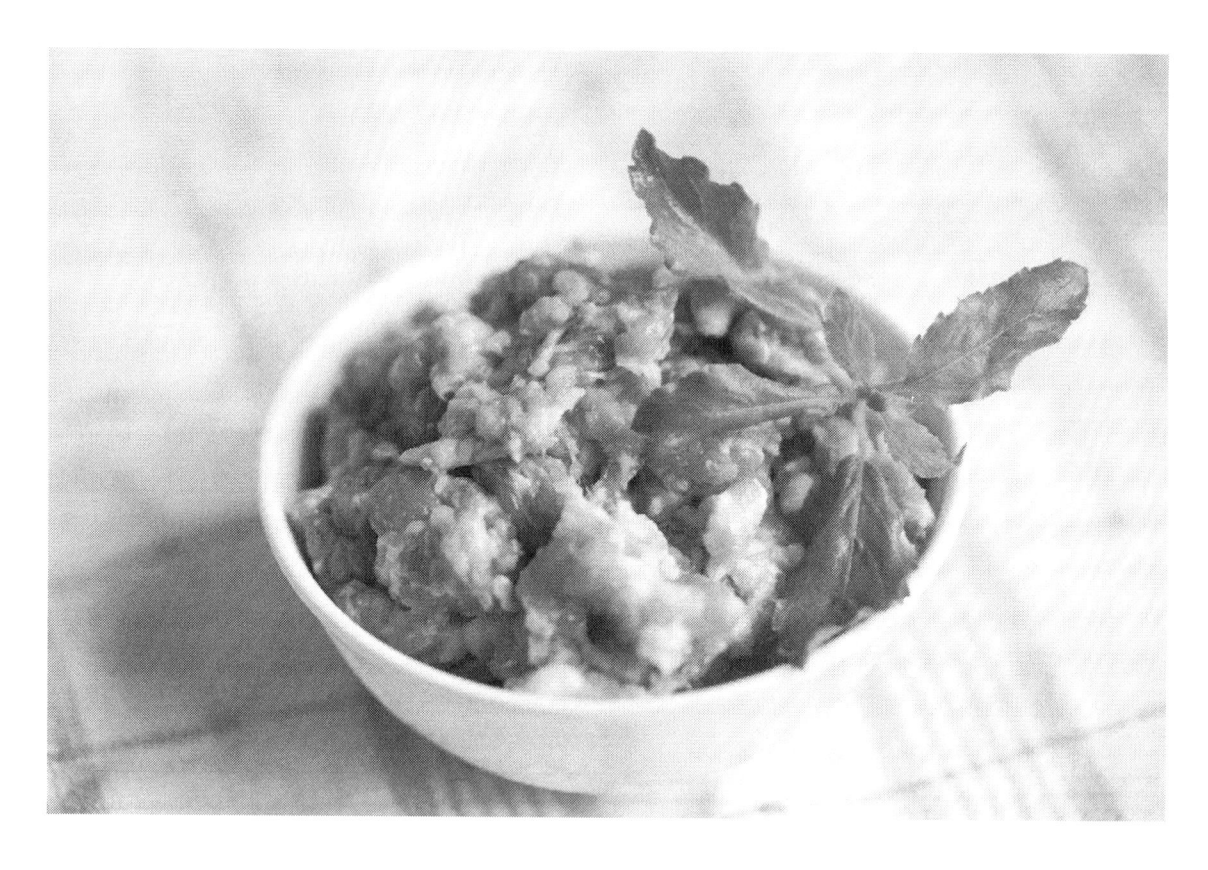

This bariatric-friendly recipe is easy to make and even kids love it. You can substitute preferred ingredients, as long as they are still healthy.

Makes 9 Servings

Cooking + Prep Time: 1 hour & 5 minutes

Ingredients:

- 1 pound of turkey, ground
- 1 diced zucchini, small
- 1 diced small onion, yellow
- 1 minced clove of garlic
- 1 pkg. of seasoning mix, taco flavor
- 1 x 10-ounce can of drained, rinsed black beans
- 8 ounces of canned refried beans, fat-free
- 8 ounces of canned tomatoes with chilies
- 2 cups of cheese blend, Mexican

Instructions:

Preheat the oven to 350F.

Spray pan with cooking spray. Set on med. heat and allow to heat up.

Sauté the vegetables with minced garlic till they soften. Drain off excess liquid, if any. Transfer to large-sized bowl.

Brown the ground meal and drain. Transfer to same bowl. Mix with tomatoes, chilies and canned beans.

Add taco seasoning mix and blend well. Transfer the mixture into 13" x 9" baking dish.

Spread out the refried beans on top of baking dish mixture. You can microwave them first if you like, to make this step easier.

Top casserole with the cheese. Bake in 350F oven for 25-35 minutes, till cheese is melty and browned a bit.

Remove baking dish from oven and cool for 10 to 15 minutes. Slice and serve.

Bariatric Dessert Recipes

29 – Butterscotch Dessert Bars

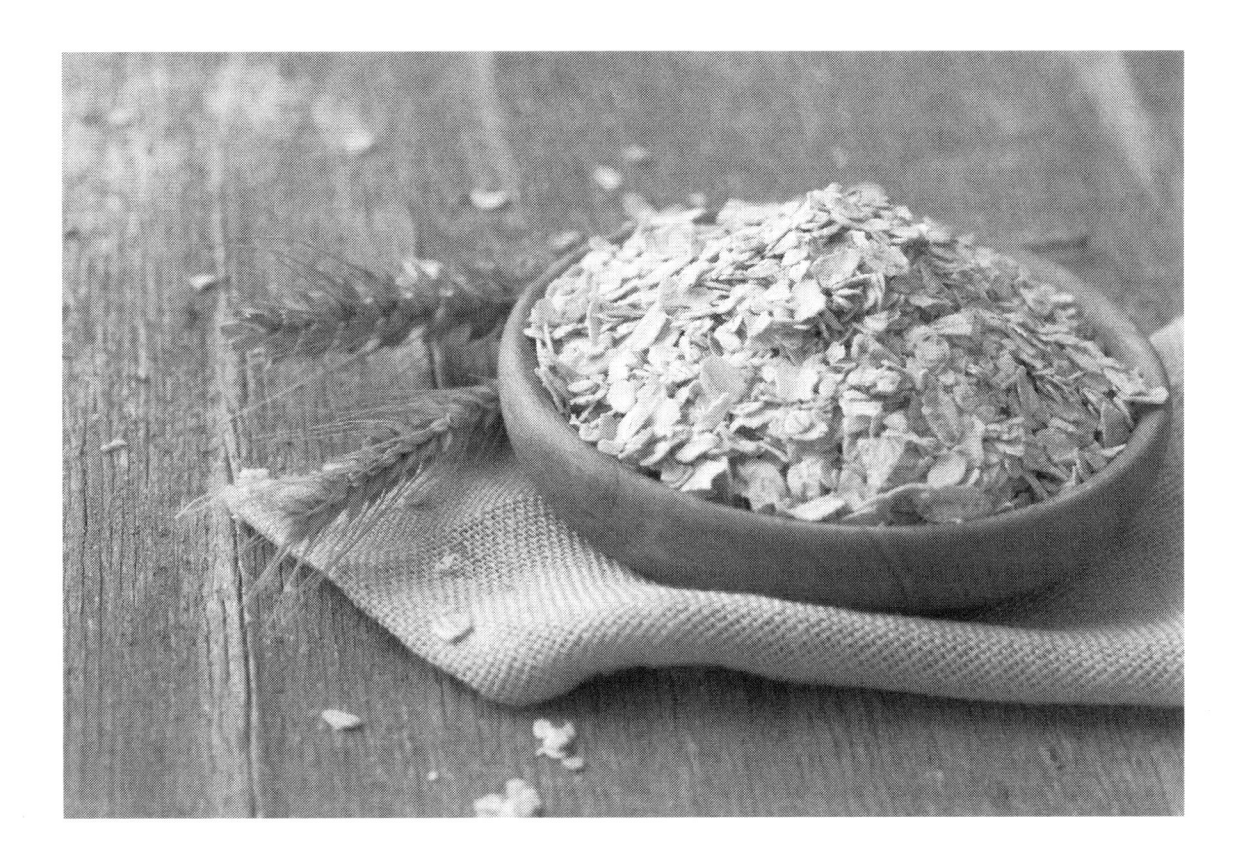

Just a small-sized square of the butterscotch bar will satisfy your craving for a sweet treat. The oats and flour are rather dry, but they make a good base for the butterscotch layer, along with a streusel-like, crumbly topping.

Makes 36 Servings

Cooking + Prep Time: 1 hour & 10 minutes

Ingredients:

- 1 cup of brown sugar, packed
- 5 tbsp. of melted butter, unsalted
- 1 tsp. of vanilla extract, pure
- 1 lightly beaten egg, large
- 9 oz. of flour, all-purpose
- 2 & 1/2 cup of oats, quick-cooking
- 1/2 tsp. + .13 tsp. of salt, kosher
- 1/2 tsp. of baking soda
- Non-stick spray
- 3/4 cup of condensed milk, sweetened, fat-free
- 1 & 1/4 cups of morsels, butterscotch
- 1/2 cup of toasted walnuts, chopped finely

Instructions:

Preheat the oven to 350F.

Combine butter and sugar in large mixing bowl. Stir in egg and vanilla. Spoon the flour lightly into dry measuring cup and level with knife.

Combine oats, flour, 1/2 tsp. of salt & baking soda in medium bowl. Add this mixture to the butter & sugar mixture. Stir till crumbly but combined.

Place three cups of the oat mixture in bottom of 13" x 9" casserole dish sprayed with non-stick spray. Press in bottom of dish. Set dish aside.

Place butterscotch morsels, condensed milk & 1/8 tsp. of salt in heavy glass bowl. Place in microwave for a minute on high setting till morsels have melted, and stir every 20 seconds or so.

Add walnuts and stir. Scrape the mixture into 13" x 9" dish and spread crust over evenly. Sprinkle remainder of oat mixture in evenly. Press into the butterscotch mixture.

Bake in 350F oven for 1/2 hour, till topping turns golden brown in color. Place dish on cooling rack. Cool fully and then serve.

30 – Cinnamon Pear

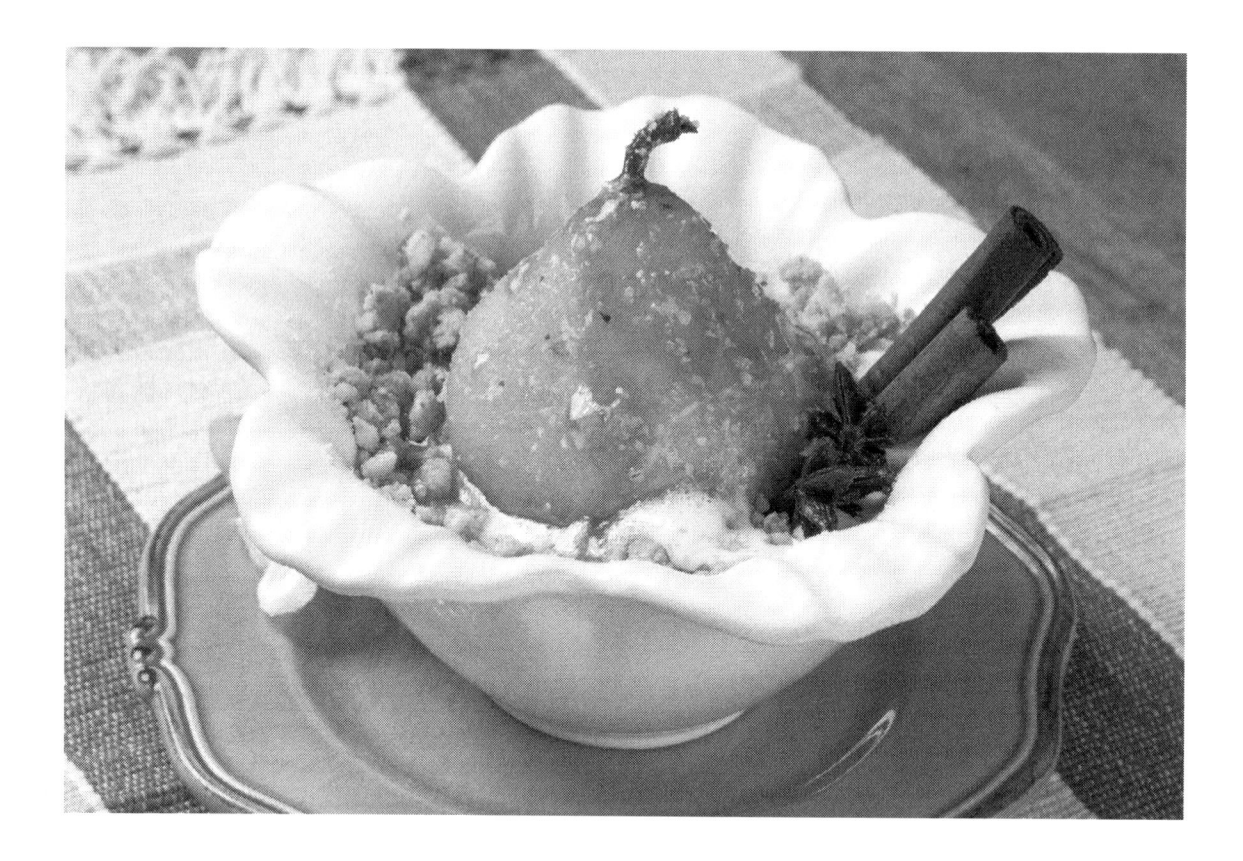

This pear makes two servings, but you can make the leftover into breakfast for the next morning. Or, it makes another delicious dessert the next day, too.

Makes 1-2 Servings

Cooking + Prep Time: 25 minutes

Ingredients:

- 1 pear, Bosc
- 1 tsp. of oil, coconut
- 1/2 cup of cottage cheese, 2%
- A dash cinnamon, ground

Instructions:

Preheat the oven to 425F.

Slice pear into halves. Remove center and seeds.

Place on cookie sheet lined with baking paper. Cook in 425F oven for 12-15 minutes. Remove. Brush top with 1 tsp. oil.

Replace in oven. Cook for 10 minutes more.

Remove from oven. Add 1/4 cup of cottage cheese to each half and sprinkle top with cinnamon. Serve.

31 – Berry Cobbler

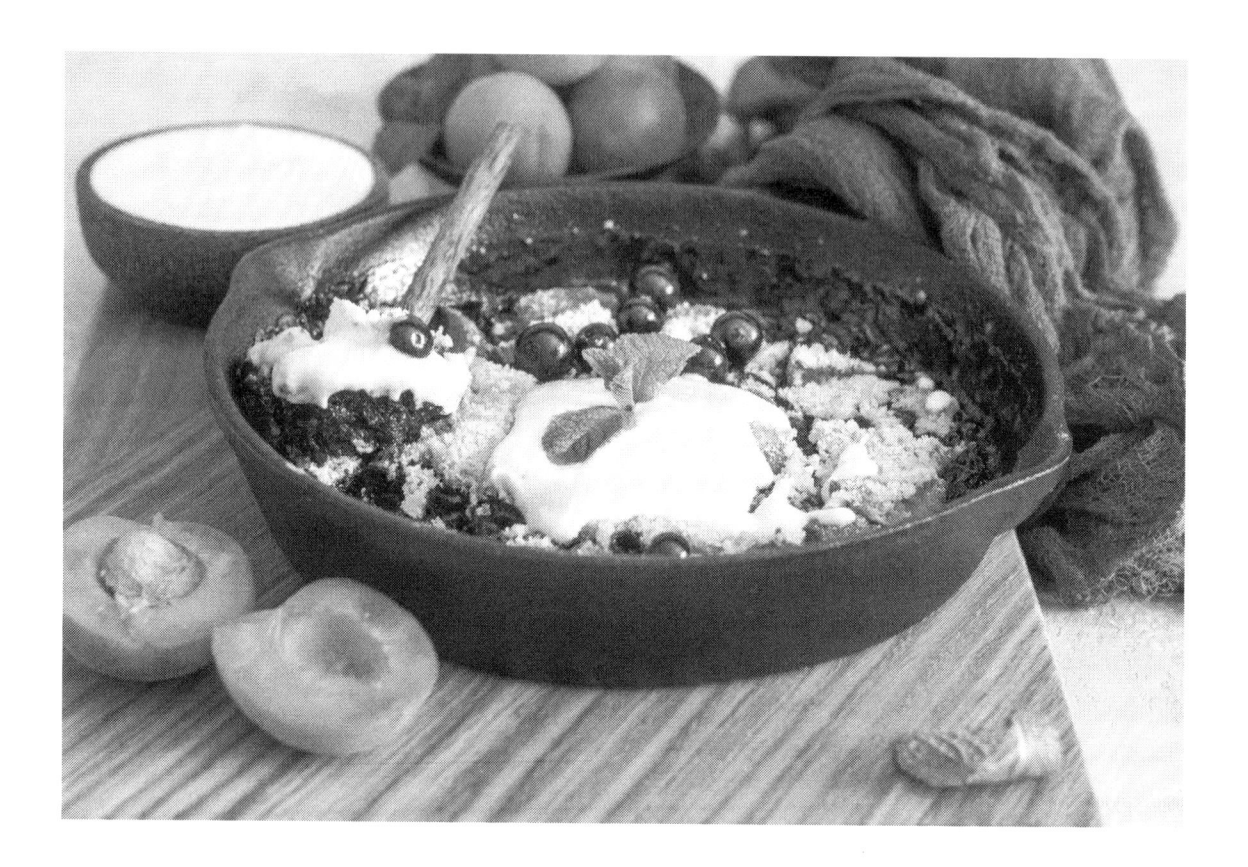

This recipe allows your slow cooker to do all the work. A muffin mix made with whole grains will create an even healthier dessert.

Makes 12 Servings

Cooking + Prep Time: 20 minutes + 4 hours slow cooker time

Ingredients:

- 1 x 14-oz. pkg. of frozen berries, mixed, packed loosely
- 1 x 21-oz. can of pie filling, blueberry
- 2 tbsp. of sugar, granulated
- 1 x 6 & 1/2-oz. pkg. of muffin mix, blueberry
- 1/3 cup of water, filtered
- 2 tbsp. of oil, vegetable

Instructions:

Spray your slow cooker lightly with non-stick spray.

Combine the frozen mixed berries, sugar and pie filling in slow cooker.

Cover slow cooker. Cook using low setting for three hours. Turn to high setting.

In medium mixing bowl, combine water, oil and muffin mix. Stir till barely combined. Spoon over the berry mixture.

Cover slow cooker. Cook for an hour on high till you can insert a toothpick in middle and have it come back clean. Turn cooker off.

Leave uncovered and cool for 30-45 minutes on wire rack. Serve.

32 – Peanut Butter Bites

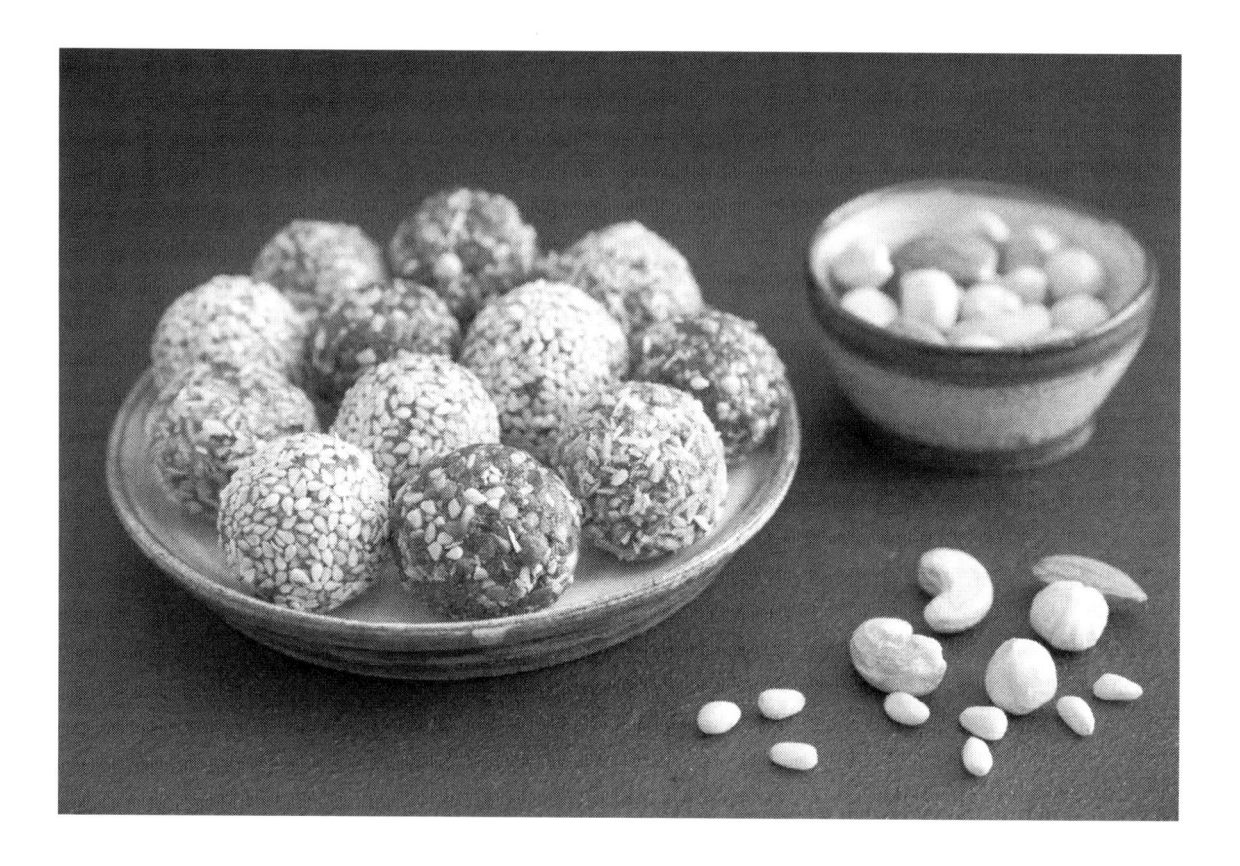

Like the remainder of these recipes, this is suited for the regular phase after bariatric surgery. You can prepare them over the weekend and snack on them all week.

Makes Various # of Servings

Cooking + Prep Time: 10 minutes

Ingredients:

- 1/4 cup of packed dates, pitted
- 1 can of drained, rinsed black beans
- 2 scoops of chocolate protein powder, vegan
- 1/4 cup peanut butter, natural
- 1/2 tsp. of salt, sea
- 1 tbsp. of powder, cacao

Instructions:

Line cookie sheet with baking paper.

Combine the dates, beans, protein powder, sea salt, peanut butter & cacao powder in food processor. Process till smooth.

Roll dough in 1" balls. Place on cookie sheet. You'll have 15-20 balls.

Place in refrigerator or freezer to firm the balls up. Serve.

33 – Skinny Brownies

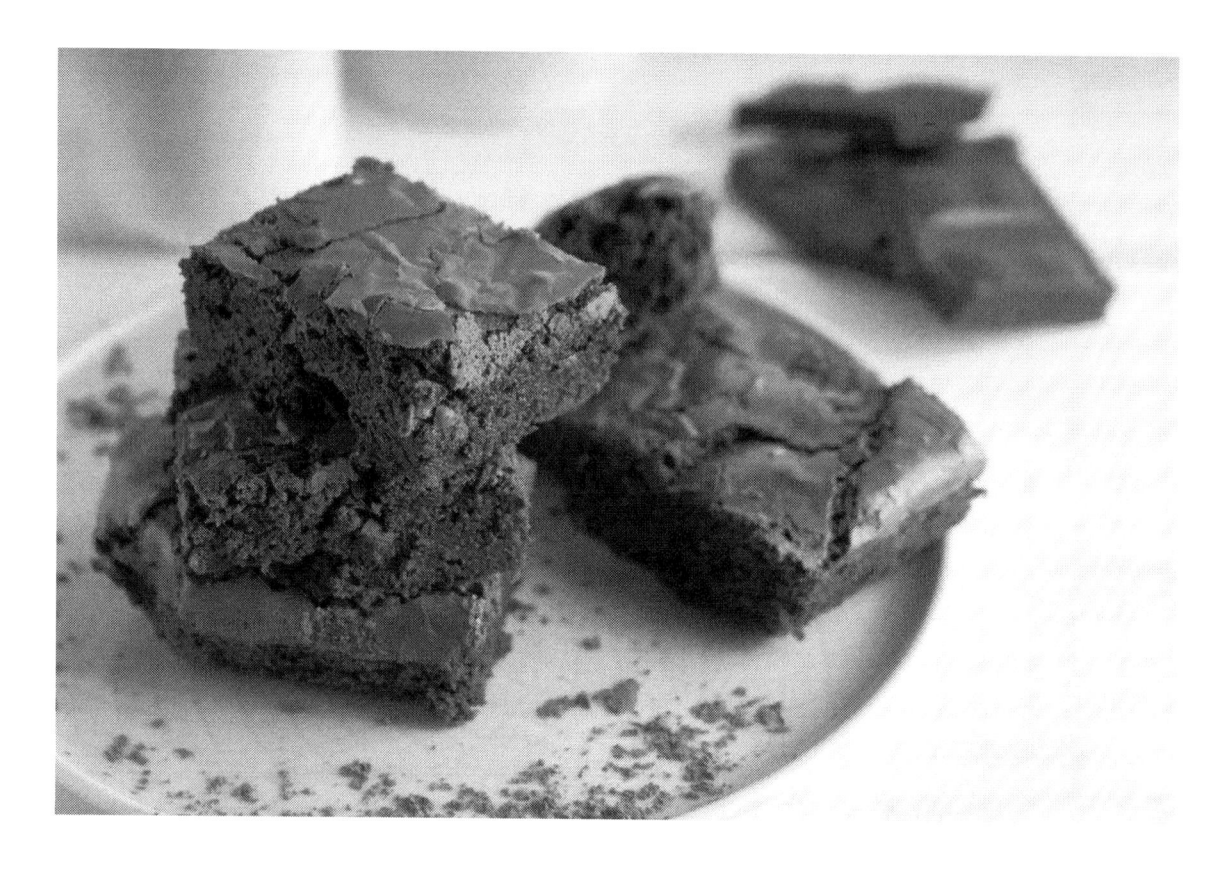

These delectable brownies contain fewer than 100 calories and they only take a minute in the microwave to prepare. They have a soft, moist, incredible taste.

Makes 1 Serving

Cooking + Prep Time: 5 minutes

Ingredients:

- 1 tbsp. of cocoa powder, unsweetened
- 2 pkts. of natural sweetener (Truvia, Stevia, etc.)
- 2 tbsp. of flour, all-purpose or almond
- 3 tbsp. of milk, almond

Instructions:

Place ingredients all in ceramic mug. Mix with whisk or fork.

Place in microwave for 1 minute on high setting. Serve warm.

Conclusion

This bariatric cookbook has shown you…

How to use different ingredients to affect unique tastes in many weight loss dishes.

How can you include phase 4 recipes in your home repertoire?

You can…

Make breakfast fritters and lime & avocado omelets, which you may not have heard of before. They are just as tasty as they sound.

Cook soups and stews, which are widely served after bariatric surgery. Find ingredients in meat & produce or frozen food sections of your local grocery store.

Enjoy making the delectable bariatric seafood dishes, including salmon and flounder. Fish is a mainstay in recipes year-round, and there are SO many ways to make it great.

Make dishes using potatoes and pasta in moderation. There is something about them that makes the dishes more comforting.

Make all kinds of bariatric desserts like peanut butter bites and berry cobbler, which will surely tempt anyone with a sweet tooth.

Enjoy these recipes with your family and friends!

About the Author

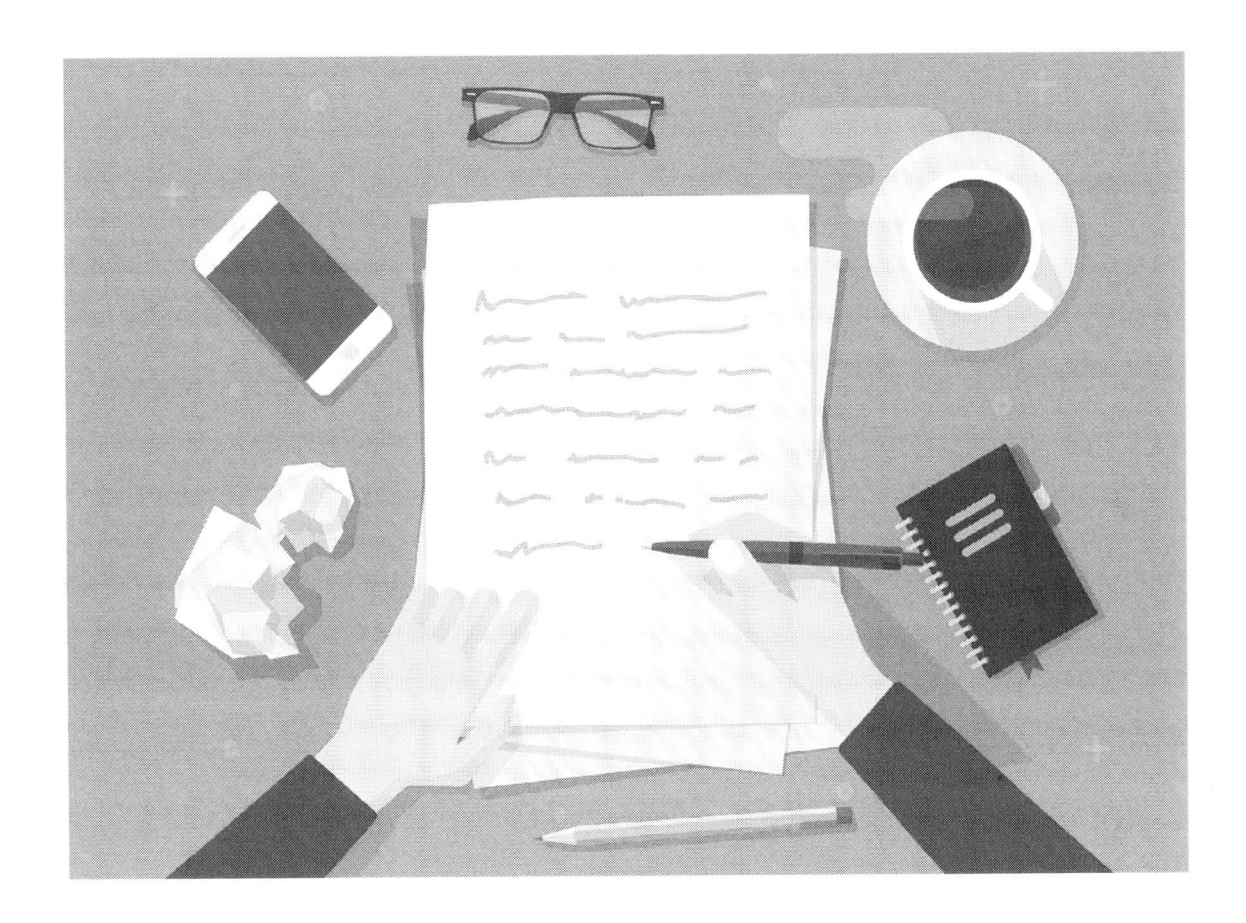

Allie Allen developed her passion for the culinary arts at the tender age of five when she would help her mother cook for their large family of 8. Even back then, her family knew this would be more than a hobby for the young Allie and when she graduated from high school, she applied to cooking school in London. It had always been a dream of the young chef to study with some of Europe's best and she made it happen by attending the Chef Academy of London.

After graduation, Allie decided to bring her skills back to North America and open up her own restaurant. After 10 successful years as head chef and owner, she decided to sell her business and pursue other career avenues. This monumental decision led Allie to her true calling, teaching. She also started to write e-books for her students to study at home for practice. She is now the proud author of several e-books and gives private and semi-private cooking lessons to a range of students at all levels of experience.

Stay tuned for more from this dynamic chef and teacher when she releases more informative e-books on cooking and baking in the near future. Her work is infused with stores and anecdotes you will love!

Author's Afterthoughts

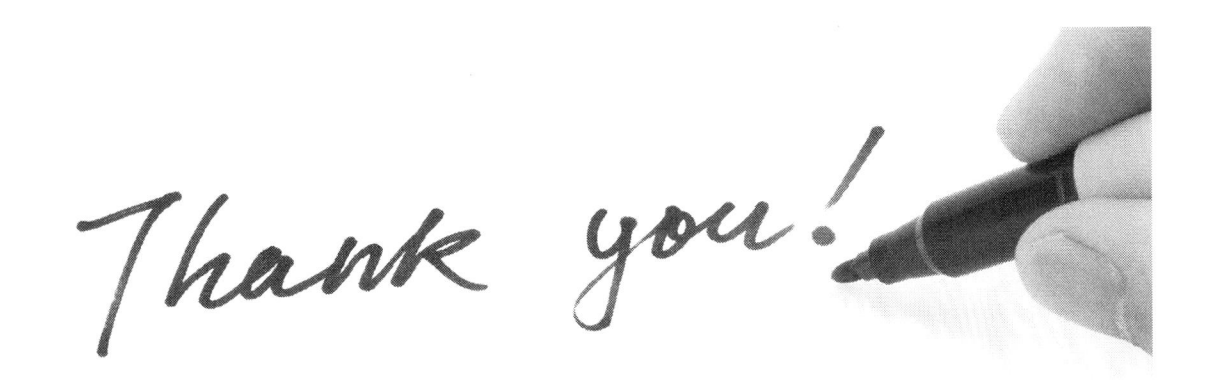

I can't tell you how grateful I am that you decided to read my book. My most heartfelt thanks that you took time out of your life to choose my work and I hope you find benefit within these pages.

There are so many books available today that offer similar content so that makes it even more humbling that you decided to buying mine.

Tell me what you thought! I am eager to hear your opinion and ideas on what you read as are others who are looking for a good book to buy. Leave a review on Amazon.com so others can benefit from your wisdom!

With much thanks,

Allie Allen